T0198195

Climate Change and Allergy

Editor

JAE-WON OH

IMMUNOLOGY AND ALLERGY CLINICS OF NORTH AMERICA

www.immunology.theclinics.com

February 2021 • Volume 41 • Number 1

ELSEVIER

1600 John F. Kennedy Boulevard • Suite 1800 • Philadelphia, Pennsylvania, 19103-2899

http://www.theclinics.com

IMMUNOLOGY AND ALLERGY CLINICS OF NORTH AMERICA Volume 41, Number 1

February 2021 ISSN 0889-8561, ISBN-13: 978-0-323-79385-8

Editor: Katerina Heidhausen
Developmental Editor: Nick Henderson

Immunology and Allergy Clinics of North America (ISSN 0889–8561) is published quarterly by Elsevier Inc., 360 Park Avenue South, New York, NY 10010-1710. Months of issue are February, May, August, and November. Periodicals postage paid at New York, NY and additional mailing offices. Subscription prices are $347.00 per year for US individuals, $827.00 per year for US institutions, $100.00 per year for US students and residents, $423.00 per year for Canadian individuals, $100.00 per year for Canadian students, $864.00 per year for Canadian institutions, $447.00 per year for international individuals, $864.00 per year for international institutions, $220.00 per year for international students. To receive student/resident rate, orders must be accompanied by name of affiliated institution, date of term, and the *signature* of program/residency coordinator on institution letterhead. Orders will be billed at individual rate until proof of status is received. Foreign air speed delivery is included in all *Clinics* subscription prices. All prices are subject to change without notice. **POSTMASTER**: Send address changes to *Immunology and Allergy Clinics of North America,* Elsevier Health Sciences Division, Subscription Customer Service, 3251 Riverport Lane, Maryland Heights, MO 63043. **Customer Service: 1-800-654-2452 (U.S. and Canada); 314-447-8871 (outside U.S. and Canada). Fax: 314-447-8029. E-mail: journalscustomerservice-usa@elsevier.com (for print support); journalsonlinesupport-usa@elsevier.com (for online support).**

Reprints. For copies of 100 or more, of articles in this publication, please contact the Commercial Reprints Department, Elsevier Inc., 360 Park Avenue South, New York, New York 10010-1710. Tel. 212-633-3874, Fax: 212-633-3820, E-mail: reprints@elsevier.com.

Immunology and Allergy Clinics of North America is covered in MEDLINE/PubMed (Index Medicus), Current Contents/Life Sciences, Science Citation Index, ISI/BIOMED, Chemical Abstracts, and EMBASE/Excerpta Medica.

Printed in the United States of America.

Contributors

EDITOR

JAE-WON OH, MD, PhD, FAAAAI
Department of Pediatrics, Hanyang University Guri Hospital, College of Medicine,
Hanyang University, Seoul, Korea

AUTHORS

PAUL J. BEGGS, PhD
Department of Earth and Environmental Sciences, Faculty of Science and Engineering,
Macquarie University, Sydney, New South Wales, Australia

DILYS BERMAN, PhD
Allergy and Immunology Unit, University of Cape Town Lung Institute, Cape Town, South
Africa

LEONARD BIELORY, MD
Professor, Center of Environmental Prediction, Rutgers University, Professor of Medicine,
Allergy, Immunology, and Ophthalmology, Hackensack Meridian School of Medicine at
Seton Hall University, Springfield, New Jersey, USA

YOUNG-JIN CHOI, MD, PhD
Clinical Professor, Department of Pediatrics, Hanyang University Guri Hospital, Guri,
Gyunggi-Do, Korea

JANET M. DAVIES, PhD
School of Biomedical Science, Queensland University of Technology, Office of Research,
Metro North Hospital and Health Service, Herston, Queensland, Australia

JEFFREY G. DEMAIN, MD, FAAAAI
Allergy Asthma and Immunology Center of Alaska, Clinical Professor, Department of
Pediatrics, University of Washington, Seattle, Washington, USA

MAE JA HAN, MS
High Impact Weather Research Department, National Institute of Meteorological
Sciences, Guri, Korea

CONSTANCE H. KATELARIS, MBBS, PhD, FRACP
Professor, Immunology and Allergy, Western Sydney University; Head of Unit,
Campbelltown Hospital, Sydney, New South Wales, Australia

KYU RANG KIM, PhD
High Impact Weather Research Department, National Institute of Meteorological
Sciences, Gangneung-si, Gangwon-do, Korea

REIKO KISHIKAWA, MD, PhD
Department of Allergology, National Hospital Organization Fukuoka National Hospital,
Fukuoka, Japan

EIKO KOTO
Assistant Clinical Research Institute of National Hospital Organization, Department of Allergology, National Hospital Organization Fukuoka National Hospital, Fukuoka, Japan

KYUNG SUK LEE, MD, PhD
Assistant Professor, Department of Pediatrics, Hanyang University Guri Hospital, Guri, Gyunggi-Do, Korea; Department of Pediatrics, College of Medicine, Hanyang University, Seoul, Korea

CHANDNI MATHUR, PhD
Ghaziabad, Uttar Pradesh, India

JAE-WON OH, MD, PhD, FAAAAI
Department of Pediatrics, Hanyang University Guri Hospital, College of Medicine, Hanyang University, Seoul, Korea

RUBY PAWANKAR, MD, PhD
Department of Pediatrics, Nippon Medical School, Tokyo, Japan

JONNY PETER, MD, PhD
Division of Allergy and Clinical Immunology, Department of Medicine, Groote Schuur Hospital, University of Cape Town, Allergy and Immunology Unit, University of Cape Town Lung Institute, Cape Town, South Africa

JILL A. POOLE, MD
Professor, Department of Medicine, Division of Allergy and Immunology, University of Nebraska Medical Center, Omaha, Nebraska, USA

GERMÁN DARÍO RAMÓN, MD, FAAAAI
Hospital Italiano Regional DelSur, Bahía Blanca, Buenos Aires, Argentina

ANDREW RORIE, MD
Assistant Professor, Department of Medicine, Division of Allergy and Immunology, University of Nebraska Medical Center, Omaha, Nebraska, USA

DIVYA SETH, MD
Assistant Professor–Clinical Educator, Division of Allergy/Immunology, Department of Pediatrics, Children's Hospital of Michigan, Wayne State University School of Medicine, Detroit, Michigan, USA

ANAND BAHADUR SINGH, PhD
Former Scientist (Emeritus), CSIR-Institute of Genomics and Integrative Biology, University Campus, Delhi, India

JIU-YAO WANG, MD, PhD
Center for Allergy and Clinical Immunology Research, College of Medicine, National Cheng Kung University Hospital, Tainan, Taiwan

LEWIS H. ZISKA, PhD
Associate Professor, Mailman School of Public Health, Columbia University, New York, New York, USA

Contents

Preface: The Impact of Climate Change on Allergy in a Changing World   ix

Jae-Won Oh

Global Climate Change and Pollen Aeroallergens: A Southern Hemisphere
Perspective   1

Janet M. Davies, Dilys Berman, Paul J. Beggs, Germán Darío Ramón, Jonny Peter,
Constance H. Katelaris, and Lewis H. Ziska

> Climatic change will have an impact on production and release of pollen, with consequences for the duration and magnitude of seasonal aeroallergen exposure and allergic diseases. Evaluations of pollen aerobiology in the southern hemisphere have been limited by resourcing and the density of monitoring sites. This review emphasizes inconsistencies in pollen monitoring methods and metrics used globally. Research should consider unique southern hemisphere biodiversity, climate, plant distributions, standardization of pollen aerobiology, automation, and environmental integration. For both hemispheres, there is a clear need for better understanding of likely influences of climate change and comprehending their impact on pollen-related health outcomes.

Allergenic Pollen Season Variations in the Past Two Decades Under Changing
Climate in the United States   17

Divya Seth and Leonard Bielory

> Prevalence of allergic diseases has been increasing due to multiple factors, among which climate change has had the most impact. Climate factors increase production of pollen, which also exhibits increased allergenicity. Also, as a result of climate change, there has been a shift in flowering phenology and pollen initiation causing prolonged pollen exposure. Various numerical models have been developed to understand the effect of climate change on pollen emission and transport and the impact on allergic airway diseases.

Climate Change and Pollen Allergy in India and South Asia   33

Anand Bahadur Singh and Chandni Mathur

> Increased levels of CO_2 and various greenhouse gases cause global warming and, in combination with pollutants from fossil fuel combustion and vehicular and industrial emissions, have been driving increases in non-communicable diseases across the globe, resulting a higher mortality and morbidity. Respiratory diseases and associated allergenic manifestations have increased worldwide, with rates higher in developing countries. Pollen allergy serves as a model for studying the relationship between air pollution and respiratory disorders. Climate changes affect the quality and amount of airborne allergenic pollens, and pollutants alter their allergenicity, resulting in greater health impacts, especially in sensitized individuals.

Climate Change and Extreme Weather Events in Australia: Impact on Allergic Diseases   53

Constance H. Katelaris

> Several climate change–related predictions and observations have been documented for the Australian continent. Extreme weather events such as cycles of severe drought and damaging flooding are occurring with greater frequency and have a severe impact on human health. Two specific aspects of climate change affecting allergic and other respiratory disorders are outlined: firstly, the consequences of extreme weather events and secondly, the change in distribution of airborne allergens that results from various climate change factors.

Climate Change, Air Pollution, and Biodiversity in Asia Pacific and Impact on Respiratory Allergies   63

Ruby Pawankar and Jiu-Yao Wang

> Allergic diseases are increasing globally. Air pollution, climate change, and reduced biodiversity are major threats to human health with detrimental effects on chronic noncommunicable diseases. Outdoor and indoor air pollution and climate change are increasing. Asia has experienced rapid economic growth, a deteriorating environment, and an increase in allergic diseases to epidemic proportions. Air pollutant levels in Asian countries are substantially higher than in developed countries. Moreover, industrial, traffic-related, and household biomass combustion and indoor pollutants from chemicals and tobacco are major sources of air pollutants. We highlight the major components of pollutants and their impacts on respiratory allergies.

The Role of Extreme Weather and Climate-Related Events on Asthma Outcomes   73

Andrew Rorie and Jill A. Poole

> Extreme weather and climate events are likely to increase in frequency and severity as a consequence of global climate change. These are events that can include flooding rains, prolonged heat waves, drought, wildfires, hurricanes, severe thunderstorms, tornadoes, storm surge, and coastal flooding. It is important to consider these events as they are not merely meteorologic occurrences but are linked to our health. We aim to address how these events are interconnected with asthma outcomes associated with thunderstorm asthma, pollen production, mold infestation from flooding events, and poor air quality during wildfires.

Insect Migration and Changes in Venom Allergy due to Climate Change   85

Jeffrey G. Demain

> Insects are highly successful animals. They have limited ability to regulate their temperature and therefore will expand range in response to warming temperatures. Climate change and associated rising global temperature is impacting the range and distribution of stinging insects. There is evidence that many species are expanding range toward the poles, primarily in response to warming. With expanded distribution of stinging insects, increased interaction with humans is anticipated with consequently increased rates of sting-related reactions and need for intervention. This

article focuses on evidence that insects are expanding their range in response to warming temperature, increasing likelihood of human interaction.

The Impact of Climate Change on Pollen Season and Allergic Sensitization to Pollens   97

Young-Jin Choi, Kyung Suk Lee, and Jae-Won Oh

Pollens are a major cause of seasonal allergic diseases. Weather may alter the production of pollens. Increased atmospheric temperatures lead to earlier pollination of many plants and longer duration of pollination, resulting in extended pollen seasons, with early spring or late winter. Longer pollen seasons increase duration of exposure, resulting in more sensitization, and higher pollen concentrations may lead to more severe symptoms. Climate changes in contact to pollens may affect both allergic sensitization and symptom prevalence with severity. The future consequences of climate change, however, are speculative, because the influence on humans, is complex.

Effect of Climate Change on Allergenic Airborne Pollen in Japan   111

Reiko Kishikawa and Eiko Koto

In Japan, the representative allergenic airborne pollen-related allergic diseases include Cupressaceae in early spring, the birch family and grass in spring and mugwort in autumn. As a result of a long- term survey the past 27 to 33 years, an increasing in the amount of conifer airborne pollen and an earlier start dispersal were observed, related climate change. In addition, an increase in the number of patients with Japanese cedar pollinosis and the severity has been observed. Provision of medical pollen information, medication and sublingual immunotherapy have all been enhanced. Recently, pollen-food allergic syndrome has become of increased interest.

Forecast for Pollen Allergy: A Review from Field Observation to Modeling and Services in Korea   127

Kyu Rang Kim, Mae Ja Han, and Jae-Won Oh

Pollen, a major causal agent of respiratory allergy, is mainly affected by weather conditions. In Korea, pollen and weather data are collected by the national observation network. Forecast models and operational services are developed and provided based on the national pollen data base. Using the pollen risk forecast information will help patients with respiratory allergy to improve their lives. Changes in temperature and CO_2 concentration by climate change affect the growth of plants and their capacity of producing more allergenic pollens, which should be considered in making the future strategy on treating allergy patients.

IMMUNOLOGY AND ALLERGY CLINICS OF NORTH AMERICA

FORTHCOMING ISSUES

May 2021
Food Allergy
Amal Assa'ad, *Editor*

August 2021
Skin Allergy
Susan T. Nedorost, *Editor*

RECENT ISSUES

November 2020
Biologics for the Treatments of Allergic Diseases
Lanny Rosenwasser, *Editor*

August 2020
Immunodeficiencies
Mark Ballow and Elena Perez, *Editors*

SERIES OF RELATED INTEREST

Medical Clinics
http://medical.theclinics.com/

THE CLINICS ARE AVAILABLE ONLINE!
Access your subscription at:
www.theclinics.com

Preface

The Impact of Climate Change on Allergy in a Changing World

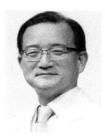

Jae-Won Oh, MD, PhD, FAAAAI
Editor

Most of the observed increase in recently global average temperatures is very likely due to the observed increase in anthropogenic greenhouse gas concentrations. Moreover, changes are also occurring in the amount, intensity, frequency, and type of precipitation as well as the increase of extreme weather events, such as droughts, thunderstorms, floods, and hurricanes.

The major changes to our world involve the atmosphere and its associated climate, including global warming induced by human activity, and are causing an impact on the biosphere, biodiversity, and the human environment. Observational evidence indicates that recent regional changes in climate, particularly increases in temperature, have already affected a diverse set of physical and biological systems in many parts of the world.

Climate change represents a massive threat to global health that could affect many disease factors in the twenty-first century. Among others, climate change influences the development of asthma and allergic respiratory diseases and also pollen and mold productions that induce allergic manifestations.

The influence of a changing climate on allergic disease has generated interest from the public and the scientific community. Climate change is a constant process that affects allergy. The climate is constantly changing and variable over time and is dependent on incoming solar radiation, outgoing thermal radiation, and the composition of the atmosphere on earth. There are multiple interrelated, potential consequences of climatic change on respiratory allergic disease. Therefore, the change can subsequently influence the occurrence of allergic diseases, such as asthma, allergic rhinitis, allergic conjunctivitis, and even atopic dermatitis.

The exact future consequences of these trends are speculative, but the allergy community should be knowledgeable about the issues, understand the effect on allergy and asthma, and be well versed in possible means to mitigate adverse health

Immunol Allergy Clin N Am 41 (2021) ix–x
https://doi.org/10.1016/j.iac.2020.10.001
0889-8561/21/© 2020 Published by Elsevier Inc.

immunology.theclinics.com

consequences. Ultimately, the approach to climate change should be integrated and anticipatory to protect and treat our patients with asthma and other allergic and climate-sensitive diseases from constituents that are likely driving this phenomenon.

This special issue was designed not only to review the clinical aspect of multifaceted allergy with diverse information of climate change in the world but also to discuss the mechanism of those phenomena.

Jae-Won Oh, MD, PhD, FAAAAI
Department of Pediatrics
Hanyang University Guri Hospital
153 Gyunchun-Ro, Guri
Gyunggi-Do 11923, Korea

E-mail address:
jaewonoh@hanyang.ac.kr

Global Climate Change and Pollen Aeroallergens

A Southern Hemisphere Perspective

Janet M. Davies, PhD[a,b,*], Dilys Berman, PhD[c], Paul J. Beggs, PhD[d],
Germán Darío Ramón, MD[e], Jonny Peter, MD, PhD[f,g],
Constance H. Katelaris, MBBS, PhD, FRACP[h], Lewis H. Ziska, PhD[i]

KEYWORDS

- Aeroallergens • Carbon dioxide • Climate change • Biodiversity

KEY POINTS

- Climate change is having an impact on pollen distributions and aeroallergen seasonal exposure globally.
- Distinctions in anthropogenic climate change between hemispheres and unique plant biogeography suggest that the southern hemisphere aeroallergen biology and clinical consequences differ from those of the northern hemisphere.
- Directions that could aid research to better monitor and evaluate climate shifts and aerobiology in the southern hemisphere are suggested.

INTRODUCTION

Pollen proteins can act as antigens for the human immune system and are capable of exacerbating allergic rhinoconjunctivitis (pollinosis) and allergic asthma. Allergic reactions are mediated by aberrant overproduction by the immune system of allergen-specific IgE that trigger an inflammatory response on re-exposure to the eliciting substance. Exposures to pollen aeroallergens are seasonal. For the southern hemisphere,

[a] School of Biomedical Science, Queensland University of Technology, Herston, Queensland 4006, Australia; [b] Office of Research, Metro North Hospital and Health Service, Herston, Queensland 4006, Australia; [c] Allergy and Immunology Unit, University of Cape Town Lung Institute, Cape Town 7700, South Africa; [d] Department of Earth and Environmental Sciences, Faculty of Science and Engineering, Macquarie University, Sydney, New South Wales 2109, Australia; [e] Hospital Italiano Regional DelSur, Bahía Blanca, Buenos Aires, Argentina; [f] Division of Allergy and Clinical Immunology, Department of Medicine, Groote Schuur Hospital, University of Cape Town, 7700 | PO Box 34560, 7937, South Africa; [g] Allergy and Immunology Unit, University of Cape Town Lung Institute, George Street, Cape Town, South Africa; [h] Western Sydney University and Campbeltown Hospital, Sydney, Australia; [i] Mailman School of Public Health, Columbia University, New York, NY 10032, USA
* Corresponding author.
E-mail address: j36.davies@qut.edu.au

Immunol Allergy Clin N Am 41 (2021) 1–16
https://doi.org/10.1016/j.iac.2020.09.002
0889-8561/21/© 2020 Elsevier Inc. All rights reserved.

immunology.theclinics.com

depending on climatic region, trees may contribute to pollen in late winter to early spring; grasses from several subfamilies dominate throughout spring into summer and autumn, and weeds contribute in summer and autumn. Health impacts of pollen allergy can be significant; approximately 10% to 40% of the global population is affected by allergic rhinitis due to seasonal pollen exposure.[1,2] Allergic diseases are increasingly recognized as one of the most prevalent and important noncommunicable diseases worldwide.[3]

Given the known influential effects of weather and climate on plant phenology and pollen per se, and the subsequent health impacts, the consequences of projected environmental and climatic changes on aeroallergen production are likely to be significant. Yet, although the sources and physical consequences of greenhouse gas emissions on weather and climate have been well reviewed,[4] the potential linkages related to seasonality of pollen exposure, magnitude of pollen production, pollen allergenicity, and thresholds of pollen exposure that lead to allergic diseases are still under investigation.

One of the most fundamental factors influencing pollen biology is temperature. Although "global warming" is generally interpreted as an average increase in surface temperature, differential increases in surface temperatures are occurring. In general, these differential temperature increases are occurring because of the relative concentration of water vapor, an important greenhouse gas. For example, in the tropics, where water vapor (humidity) is an important greenhouse gas, rising levels of carbon dioxide (CO_2), another greenhouse gas, are not expected to result in as great an increase in surface temperature, as in regions where the air is dry (ie, less water vapor).[5] Hence, observed changes in surface temperature are greater at the poles and desert areas, where water vapor is low.

Such geographic changes, large and small, in daily and seasonal temperatures will have obvious biological consequences for floral phenology and pollen release. Shifts in phenology are among the most consistent findings in studies of global climate change and warming temperatures.[6,7] Such shifts, in turn, will affect the timing and duration of flowering with consequences for both pollen production and seasonal exposure. Climatic studies also suggest that extreme heat and precipitation events are likely to increase in frequency, intensity, and duration in coming decades in response to changing climate, potentially exacerbating pollen and fungal spore season duration and exposure.[8]

A second, more obscure link to pollen biology is that CO_2, in addition to being a greenhouse gas, is the singular supplier of carbon for photosynthesis and plant growth. At present, more than 90% of all plant species (including all tree species) function below the optimal CO_2 concentration needed to maximize growth and reproduction; consequently, the rapid increase in atmospheric CO_2, in addition to its role in climate change, likely will stimulate growth and flower production of many known allergenic plants. At present, there also is limited evidence that rising CO_2 concentrations also may advance flowering time, although the degree of advancement appears to be species specific.[9,10]

Although Whilst additional information is needed, there is a clear prospective association between climatic change, aerobiology, and allergic disease.[11] It seems likely that ongoing changes in CO_2 concentration, temperature, and other climate variables will intensify these associations, especially in regard to seasonality of pollen exposure and amount of pollen produced by a given plant species during a season.

A HEMISPHERIC PERSPECTIVE

Currently, the foremost locus of research regarding climate change and pollen aerobiology has been in the northern hemisphere, primarily in North America and Europe.

But how relevant or applicable are these data to the southern hemisphere? To address this fundamental question, it is important to consider some unique geographic and biological hemispheric distinctions.

For example, increases in atmospheric CO_2 concentrations in the southern hemisphere typically trail those in the north. The higher northern hemisphere levels occur because CO_2 sources (eg, fossil fuel emissions) are higher; in addition, CO_2 sinks, such as oceans, are predominant in the southern hemisphere. Similarly, greater CO_2-induced increases in temperature are associated with greater land area relative to areas with open water as with the northern hemisphere. The greater ocean-to-land ratio in the south may be useful in understanding delayed responses to global temperature changes between northern and southern hemispheres.[12,13] In one of the longest analyses of surface temperature trends (1931–2015), however, Kruger and Nxumalo[14] note a general increase in extreme warm events and a general decrease in extreme cold events across South Africa. Changes in maximum temperatures may vary by location (as in the northern hemisphere), but there is a distinct increase in maximum temperatures across diverse locations (**Fig. 1**).

In addition to the rate of warming, there also are unique flora associated with the southern hemisphere. These flora also are capable of producing allergenic pollen; but there are prolific plant species of northern origin that have established and become widespread in the southern hemisphere. One of the most egregious is *Parthenium hysterophorus* (false ragweed or star weed) originating from northeast Mexico. *Parthenium* weed is present in South America and has been introduced to Australia. It can be toxic to animals and humans and cause hypersensitivity responses like hay fever, photodermatitis, asthma, skin rashes, peeling skin, puffy eyes, excessive water loss, swelling and itching of mouth and nose, constant cough, running nose, and eczema.[15,16]

Of particular importance to the subtropical regions of the southern hemisphere is the effect of elevated CO_2 on grass pollen. Grasses use either a 3-carbon (C_3) or 4-carbon (C_4) photosynthetic pathway. The C_4 pathway utilizes more carbon and loses less water than C_3 in the process. In the absence of deciduous trees (birch, ash, poplar, and hazel) from subtropical regions of southeast Queensland, Australia, the contribution of grass pollen to the total annual pollen load is elevated relative to northern

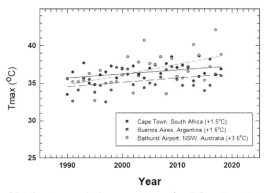

Fig. 1. Time series of highest recorded temperature for 3 locations in the southern hemisphere: Cape Town, South Africa; Buenos Aires, Argentina; and Bathurst, New South Wales, Australia. The number next to the location is the increase in maximum temperature (Tmax) recorded between 1990 and 2018.

temperate climate zones.[17] As CO_2 increases, changes in relative competition and demography are likely between C_3 temperate and C_4 tropical grasses associated with relative photosynthetic stimulation by CO_2 as well as potential changes in water loss and desiccation, suggesting that ecological niches for subtropical grasses may be altered with climate change.[18]

Grass pollens are the major cause of pollinosis in many parts of the world.[19] For South America, Panicoideae and Chloridoideae are C_4 grasses typical of tropical and subtropical arid habitats and are well represented in Argentina, Brazil, and Uruguay.[20] In seasonal climates, C_3 grasses increase in winter and flower in spring, whereas C_4 grasses grow and flower in summer and early autumn.[21] Across the continent of Australia, there is a latitudinal gradient in the distribution of subtropical C_4 and temperate C_3 grass species,[22] with Panicoideae and Chloridoideae species dominating at latitudes closer to the equator and temperate Pooideae dominating at higher latitudes with temperate climates.[23]

Climatic global change, with an increase in atmospheric CO_2 concentration and temperature, habitat transformation, and biodiversity loss, may lead to an expansion of the C_4 grasses over typical C_3 grass areas.[24,25] The change in the proportion of C_3 and C_4 grasses may, in turn, be a factor that alters the number of allergic patients.[18] Recently, it was demonstrated that subtropical grass pollens are significantly important in the skin sensitization of patients with allergic rhinitis in the city of Bahia Blanca, in southern Argentina,[26] and in South Africa[27] as well as in subtropical regions of Australia.[28] Representation of pollen allergen extracts, however, relevant to the southern hemisphere, such as for standardized subtropical grass pollens, are not all commercially available for clinical diagnosis and therapy in these regions.[21]

Although plant species, the rate of warming, and the concentration of CO_2 may vary hemispherically, the consequences, in terms of climate change, and the need to monitor subsequent changes in pollen phenology and health impact still are present. As emphasized by Haberle and colleagues,[29] aerobiology in the southern hemisphere is complex. Changes in temperature, rainfall, and the environment generally will span from the tropics to temperate zones.

SOUTHERN HEMISPHERE AEROALLERGEN MONITORING AND CLIMATE CHANGE: CHALLENGES

Regardless of location, the impacts of aeroallergens on human health are consequential. For example, allergic rhinitis affects approximately 19.3% of people in Australia[30] and approximately 26% of people in New Zealand.[31] Australia also has a high occurrence of allergy relative to a range of common and important aeroallergens.[32] Limited site-specific studies on the prevalence of sensitization to pollens in Australia, however, may not represent the complete picture of sensitization rates over the whole continent. For example, the prevalence of allergic sensitization to timothy grass pollen was 29% of 552 adults by skin prick test in Melbourne, but this grass is rare in the Victoria environment.[33] Ryegrass pollen would have been more relevant to test and although timothy and ryegrass are both temperate Pooideae grasses, there can be differences in level of allergic sensitization.[34] In Western Australia, the frequencies of serum IgE reactivity with ryegrass and Bermuda grass pollen were 41% and 36%, respectively, in a group of 1380 teenagers from an unselected birth cohort study.[35] Elsewhere, the frequency of grass pollen–positive skin prick tests in Australian school children ranged from 10% to 20%, depending on the region and the grass pollen tested.[36,37] Studies of adolescents in Cape Town, South Africa, from 1995 to 2002, indicated significant increases in asthma, allergic rhinitis, and atopic eczema.[38]

There is an existing need to monitor pollen and to determine likely or potential health outcomes of pollen exposure in diverse phytogeographical and climatic regions of the southern hemisphere. Climate change imposes another challenge: to begin to integrate and compare measurements of pollen aerobiology across southern hemisphere locations to determine current impacts and to identify countries or geographic regions that may be at greater risk. Pollen monitoring for much of the southern hemisphere (**Fig. 2**), however, remains limited to monitoring in urban areas with diverse aerobiological signatures observed in diverse biogeographical regions.[29] Few long-term (eg, decadal) attempts have been made to determine general patterns for allergen seasonality or determine variation in pollen composition.[39–41] Progress, however, is ongoing.

Since 2013, Australia has demonstrated a surge of pollen monitoring, reporting, forecasting, and research. Initial funding from the Australian Centere for Ecological Analysis and Synthesis facilitated the formation of the Australian Aerobiology Working Group, which developed into the collaboration known as AusPollen Aerobiology Collaboration Network. This collaboration has advanced understanding of pollen seasonality and diversity throughout Australia significantly.[22,23,29,42,43] A key strength of this collaboration has been its broad interdisciplinary team and transdisciplinary approach.[23,44] The team has received further support from the Australian National Health and Medical Research Council, the Australian Research Council, and the Victoria Government in response to the deadly Melbourne epidemic thunderstorm asthma event of November 21, 2016. Following this 2016 thunderstorm asthma epidemic,[45–47] the largest ever globally, a review of aerobiological, meteorologic, and individual susceptibility factors associated with thunderstorm asthma[48] was commissioned by the Victoria Department of Health and Human Services. A rapid public health response and emergency service preparedness program (https://www2.health.vic.gov.au/public-health/environmental-health/climate-weather-and-public-health/thunderstorm-asthma) was initiated, including the Victoria

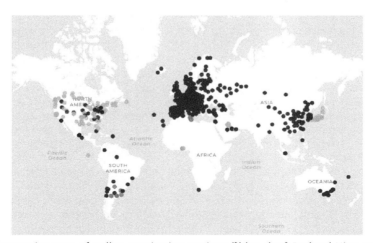

Fig. 2. Interactive map of pollen monitoring stations ([*blue dots*] Burkard Hirst traps; [*red dots*] automated; and [*orange dots*] Rotorod). Note variation in monitoring sites between hemispheres. (*From* Buters JTM, Antunes C, Galveias A, et al. Pollen and spore monitoring in the world. Clin Transl Allergy, 2018;8:9-14; with permission.)

Thunderstorm Asthma Pollen Surveillance Project managed by the Bureau of Meteorology. The AusPollen collaboration has developed an Australian Standard,[49] engaged in international collaboration,[43,50] instigated quality control exercises,[51] evaluated perceived benefits and uses of pollen information by community,[22] and integrated with other Australian (eg, AirRater, University of Tasmania) and international initiatives, such as AutoPollen and the International Association for Aerobiology.

Similarly, in South Africa, long-term pollen records only exist for Cape Town, where pollen profiles and seasonal differences have been mapped from 1984 to 2014,[52] with sporadic pollen records for other cities, such as Johannesburg and Durban.[53] In KwaZulu-Natal, a study compared fossil pollen with modern pollen to identify changes in the vegetation over time.[54] Fortunately, the situation has new impetus, with a network of pollen monitoring stations recently established in August 2019, the South African Pollen Network (SAPNET). The SAPNET team includes aeropalynologists, clinicians, climate scientists, statisticians, and air quality scientists based at 7 universities and research centers. Pollen concentrations now are measured daily in 7 cities within 6 different vegetation biomes using volumetric spore traps. Early results highlight large regional differences and have even brought the presence of the highly allergenic weed *Ambrosia artemisiifolia* (ragweed) to the attention of allergists. This is consequential, because, despite knowledge of its presence known to local plant scientists, ragweed has not been incorporated into skin prick tests or specific IgE testing panels prior to 2019.

In Argentina, attempts to develop a network of pollen monitoring through the Asociación Argentina de Alergia e Inmunologia Clinica (AAAeIC) commenced in 2006 but sustaining this network has been challenging due to economic fluctuations and limited resourcing. Despite its discontinuity, throughout these 14 years, the AAAeIC was able to monitor the pollen of almost 12 different cities with the presence of different species of pollen. Within this network, different pollen collectors, Rotorod (IQVIA, PA, USA), Burkard (Burkard Manufacturing, UK), and Lanzoni (Lanzoni SRL, Italy), have been used. The AAAeIC recently published the *Atlas Alergopalinológico de la República Argnetina*.[55] This atlas attempts to unify practical monitoring methods and offers content to develop aerobiology for the purpose of providing allergy information.

Unfortunately, at present, few attempts have been made to incorporate climatic and/or CO_2 influences on studies of aeroallergen exposures and allergic disease within the southern hemisphere.[56] Yet, it can be argued that the southern hemisphere is likely to encounter similar consequences as the north, for example, changes in the distribution of known allergenic plant taxa; changes in pollen season start date, end date, and length; changes in pollen allergenicity; and changes in seasonal pollen integral, or pollen load.

Are there lessons that can be learned from allergists, botanists, and aerobiologists in the northern hemisphere that would be of value for southern hemisphere research efforts? Yes, but as with all lessons, a value can be attached—some aspects are worth doing and others are to be avoided.

There are shortcomings in efforts to monitor pollen regardless of hemisphere. For example, there is no widespread, consistent set of guidelines for pollen collection, assessment, and reporting. Europe has advanced in recent years with the publication of a Technical Specification and now Standard for Sampling And Analysis Of Airborne Pollen Grains and Fungal Spores.[57,58] Quality control assessments of individuals involved in pollen counting from Spanish and European Union pollen monitoring networks[59] informed the AusPollen quality control assessments.[51]

Effort is being made to compile and analyze regional or continental responses that could be associated with climate change, or rising CO_2[50,60–62]; yet, such attempts remain uncoordinated and sporadic. Limitations and biases due to technical differences in collection site, instrumentation, and counting procedures are not well considered or accounted for.

Unstandardized pollen monitoring practices reflect, in part, the autonomy of allergists and pollen counters as well as inadequate financial resourcing. The independence of those who take responsibility for counting pollen is understandable. It is labor intensive and requires extensive training to identify and enumerate pollen. To do so on a continuous basis requires expertise and fortitude of character that not everyone possesses.

But such independence can be a stumbling block for cooperation. There are loose affiliations (eg, National Allergy Bureau) and business interests (eg, IQVIA) associated with training and certification of pollen identification and counting in the United States and Europe. There are few regulations or metrics, however, that are standardized across locations. How pollen is collected is site specific and can vary considerably (Rotorod, Burkard Spore Traps, and gravimetric methods), yet different sampling methods have different efficiencies,[63] and concentrations obtained by different sampling methods not always are directly comparable.[64,65] The Rotorod device may have advantages in very windy regions, such as coastal regions of Argentina, near the Atlantic, and to the south, which have significantly high average daily wind speeds (Ramón, personal communication 2020). The amount of area counted on the impaction surface (slide or Melinex tape) affects the accuracy of pollen concentration estimates but confidence intervals for pollen concentration values are not routinely provided with pollen records.[66]

In addition to different sampling methodologies, there are no consistent benchmarks used to define features of the pollen season. For some locations, the start of a pollen season can be defined when the cumulative pollen count reaches 5% and ends when it reaches 95% of the total pollen for a given year.[67] This can be referred to as the annual pollen integral (ie, seasonal pollen integral, or pollen load) or yearly cumulative count (some locations use 1% and 99% values). Aerobiology Canada uses a different seasonal definition—that of pollen persistence, that is, season is initiated with 3 days to 5 days of continuous pollen and ends with the last 3-day to 5-day period of continuous pollen. New metrics for the pollen season characteristics are emerging but none is accepted as standard, hampering comparability of reported study outcomes.[50,68,69] To be effective, globally harmonized terminology for pollen season metrics, as suggested by Pfaar and colleagues and Galan and colleagues,[68,70] need to be well communicated, adopted, and implemented.

Finally, there is a fundamental issue of the sparsity of sampling sites in the southern hemisphere. Airborne pollen concentrations are reported as if they were ubiquitously representative across a local geographic area, and few guidelines exist for interpreting them.[64] For example, there is substantial physical and biological heterogeneity within an urban landscape with consequences for spatial and seasonal variability of airborne pollen concentrations.[39] Yet, for many large urban areas, 1 or 2 rooftop pollen samplers provide pollen information for an entire city. Lack of funding, and lack of resourcing more generally, is a primary driver of the inadequate spatial density of pollen monitoring. There often is inadequate temporal coverage, with many sites unable to monitor year-round and having to stop monitoring for significant periods of time (often years) while further funding is sought.

Overall, even as rising CO_2 and climate change necessitate a greater need to assess spatial and temporal changes in pollen, and the consequences for human health, there are fundamental flaws within the current monitoring system that make meeting this challenge more difficult.

NEXT STEPS

There is no doubt that pollen monitoring has been longer and more spatially extensive in the northern hemisphere relative to the southern hemisphere (see **Fig 2**), yet it also is clear that all pollen monitoring efforts, although notable, fall short of assessing or preparing for climate change impacts. Can current efforts in the southern hemisphere to incorporate the impact of CO_2 and climate on plant biodiversity and pollen aerobiology benefit from the northern hemisphere's oversights? It can be argued that southern resources are newer, and less available; yet, it also can be maintained that adaptation is more likely for smaller groups and younger associates. If adaptation is possible, what steps should be taken?

Plant Biogeographical Diversity

There is an immediate need to understand and document the role of climate and CO_2 in changing biogeographical diversity and evolutionary potential of known allergenic plant taxa. Understandably, airborne pollen records are based on what has been observed in the past; yet, it also is evident that as climate changes, or new species are introduced, pollen sources will remain in flux. Such sources may include highly invasive species (eg, *Ambrosia* and *Parthenium*) that are significantly allergenic; alternatively, native species unique to the southern hemisphere may remain uncharacterized in regard to their contribution to allergic diseases.[36,71,72]

Observation and documentation of new (and old) pollen sources may benefit from citizen science and remote sensing as a means to maintain up-to-date biogeographical distributions.[43,73] Application of DNA meta-barcode techniques can enable documentation of pollen aerobiome diversity; however, this information only now is being applied to environmental air samples collected by cyclonic samplers or routine Hirst-style pollen and spore traps.[74,75] Yet, such information would provide valuable insight into biogeographical distribution and phenological patterns of pollen release and distribution and how these spatiotemporal patterns, in turn, respond to current and future climatic change.

Standardization of Pollen Metrics

At present, there is no uniform standard for collecting pollen. The 2 most widely applied collection methodologies, a Burkard Hirst–type volumetric pollen trap and a Rotorod volumetric sampler, can differ in their sensitivity, depending on particle size[64]; similarly, site pollen collection often is listed as rooftop, with less detail about height above ground level or surrounding vegetation. Similarly, there is no uniform standard as to what constitutes a pollen season with different groups applying different metrics. Yet, acceptance of a uniform standard would be invaluable in evaluating climate impacts. The "5%"approach to mark beginning of a pollen season can result in temporal anomalies; that is, if the total pollen accumulations for 2 consecutive years were 2000 and 5000, then the start of the season would not be noted until counts reached 100 and 250, respectively. Using this system to mark beginning and end of a pollen season would mask any season length trends associated with climate/temperature. In contrast, a consecutive day metric, as described previously, would be more sensitive to climate-induced changes in start and end times, especially if springs arrived earlier or if falls were delayed.[50]

Automation and Sampling Sites

There is an obvious need to provide relevant pollen information in the context of changing climate or population demographics (eg, city vs rural). Such a need contrasts, however, with the number of trained counters and site availability. For example, Sydney, Australia, with an estimated metropolitan population of more than 4 million, has 2 urban pollen monitoring sites.

Automated pollen monitoring using recognition software has been suggested as a means to bridge the gap. In 1 report, a comparison of a Burkard system with a fully automated image recognition–based pollen monitoring system (BAA500 Helmut Hund Gmb, Germany) for daily pollen concentrations was highly correlated (r = 0.98); however, some specific pollen sources (eg, *Salix*) were not identified satisfactorily.[76] Šaulienė and colleagues[77] have similarly evaluated the capabilities of another automated pollen monitor based on fluorometric detection. The latest innovation incorporated fluorometry and holographic image recognition.[78] Moves toward automation are accelerating rapidly, particularly in Europe, where the AutoPollen program represents large potential for progress that automatic pollen observations provide, from the actual observation through to the final end-user–defined product.[79]

Such sensors are low maintenance and do not require certified (human) pollen counters, making data comparisons across space and time more consistent. In addition, they can be disseminated in greater numbers as a means to help quantify heterogenic pollen variability. For example, urban areas typically are warmer than surrounding rural areas, with documented effects of microclimate on pollen release and load.[80] Yet, at present, there are insufficient pollen monitoring sites to document urban-rural differences in pollen exposure.

Environmental Interactions

Airborne pollen reflects current climate and flora for a given region. But anthropogenic climate change is complex, and there are likely to be other concurrent disturbances that may interact with pollen to exacerbate—or improve—human health outcomes. Climate-induced changes in temperature and rainfall will be consequential and need to be modeled and incorporated into pollen forecasts; certainly large-scale changes, such as the El Niño Southern Oscillation or Indian Ocean Dipole, should be considered.[81]

But what is the role of other climatic consequences? Australia, during the summer of 2019 to 2020, experienced an unprecedented wildfire season with significant health impacts,[82] which was exacerbated by climate change, with an estimated affected area of 110,000 km^2 (11 million hectares). How will this have an impact on the biogeography of anemophilous plant species? Could pollen levels decline? Alternatively, fires produce fine particulate pollution, known as particles that measure less than 2.5 μm across, that can be transported long distances. Such particles may exacerbate pollen sensitivity and related asthma.[83] How will concurrent changes in fire outbreaks and climate alter biodiversity, plant distributions, and pollen seasonality for Australia? Thunderstorms have been linked to asthma epidemics, especially during the grass pollen seasons.[47] Such extreme meteorologic events are projected to increase in frequency and/or severity in the future,[84,85] yet the public health consequences remain unknown.

There are, in effect, several probable means by which climate change could affect air quality; a better understanding of the risks of coexposure to both pollen and air pollutants is needed to inform and respond to likely health threats. Similarly, a more integrated approach to assessment, forecasting, and public communication of air quality, which considers the physical, chemical, and biological components and the interactions between them, is now being called for.[86]

Modeling

Understanding and documenting the complex interactions between disparate meteorologic variables, plant physiology, and their interactions with human activities (eg, air pollution and climate change) and the subsequent consequences on pollen production, seasonality, and health outcomes is a daunting task. Although individual, reductionist experiments are necessary and vital to understanding these linkages, modeling approaches to integrate physical and biological changes, especially in the context of problematic climatic shifts, will be necessary to encompass a full range of outcomes, including those related to public health.[87] Such efforts will need to incorporate myriad sources of pollen data into numerical forecast systems. Examples of these data could include phenological observations, demographic changes in plant pollen sources, and social sensing as well as data from symptom trackers or personal monitors.[88,89] Potentially, improved aeroallergen forecasts could be developed that provide detailed pollen information specific to a given population (eg, urban or rural). Overall, it is hoped that allergists, plant scientists, climatologists, and mathematicians can be encouraged to work together and assimilate their expertise for model frameworks that not only address vulnerabilities but also provide insight into research priorities, especially in regard to climate change.

SUMMARY

The relationships between weather, climate, and pollen and the resulting consequences for human health are universally acknowledged. Pollen-induced allergic rhinitis affects 10% to 40% of populations; it can predispose people to more frequent sinus infections, contribute to poor sleep quality, impair learning, and reduce productivity, and, for the people who suffer from allergic rhinitis with comorbid asthma, it can make asthma more difficult to control.[72]

Given these links, the role of ongoing environmental and climatic change on aeroallergen production and spread is likely to be substantial. Northern hemisphere efforts have provided sufficient information to confirm that climate change and/or rising CO_2 can have an impact on aeroallergen metrics, from taxa distribution to pollen production and atmospheric concentration to allergenicity, and that these changes appear to be happening in real time.[62,80] Yet, it is clear that to continue this work, coordinated multidisciplinary research involving allergists, health care professionals, ecologists, and aerobiologists is necessary for success.[23,44,48] There are both enablers and barriers, however, to multidisciplinary and intersectoral partnerships as outlined by Davies and colleagues.[23] Enablers include access to diverse skills and knowledge, amplification of productivity, influence beyond the usual arena, and incubation of new solutions to shared problems. Barriers include field specific language and concepts, time pressures, and publication challenges as well as facing autonomously managed infrastructure already in place; the lack of consistent standards for monitoring and recording pollen among locations; nonappreciation of climate change impacts; and lack of recognition or funding sources necessary to further coordination.

Better understanding of the health and socioeconomic impacts of pollen allergen exposure and associated allergic respiratory as well as other chronic inflammatory diseases is needed in relevant populations of the southern hemisphere.[90] In particular, given the unique geographic, climatic, and biological diversity of pollen aerobiomes in the southern hemisphere, understanding the clinically relevant local thresholds of pollen exposure that are associated with ocular, nasal, and lower respiratory symptoms is needed.

In summary, new opportunities for southern hemisphere research focused on standardized pollen monitoring are needed to enable the generation of long-term data sets necessary to assess broad-scale trends in pollen aerobiology with climate change. In the absence of high-density, manual pollen monitoring stations, integration of airborne pollen records with innovative landcover, and greenness indices informed by near-ground automated, fixed-site time-series digital camera photography of vegetation (phenocam) monitoring and satellite remote sensing are being applied to advance this field of research. There remains a challenge to understand and respond to the consequences of rising CO_2 and climate change on aeroallergen exposure in the southern hemisphere and the corresponding influence on allergic respiratory diseases. There are unique opportunities, and challenges, for scientists in current or emerging networks, such as the SAPNET, AAAeIC, and AusPollen, to accomplish these goals.

Threat recognition and unity of purpose, justifiable concern regarding climate change, uniform standards, cooperation, and support from governments all are necessary to address the health challenges posed by climate change, not simply those of aeroallergens and air quality. These emerging threats are of significant public concern, and it is hoped that southern nations will be able to monitor, prepare, and evaluate the effects and health impacts of climate change on pollen exposure.

CLINIC CARE POINTS

Pearls
  Climate change almost certainly will influence aeroallergen exposure seasonally and temporally throughout the southern hemisphere.
  Interactions between aeroallergens and other environmental events (thunderstorms and storms) may exacerbate existing pollen-based allergies, for example, in Australia.
  Clinical increases in aeroallergen associated illness, pollinosis, allergic rhinitis, and asthma can be anticipated.
Pitfalls
  Allergenic plant species within the southern hemisphere that may be impacted by climate and/or rising levels CO_2 have not been fully identified.
  At present, there is a need for consolidation and uniformity among southern hemisphere countries in relation to methodology, reporting, and clinical response to climate and/or CO_2-induced changes in aeroallergen biology.

DISCLOSURE

JMD leads the NHMRC AusPollen Partnership Project (GNT 1116107) with matching cash and in kind co-sponsorship from The Australasian Society for Clinical Immunology and Allergy, Asthma Australia, Bureau of Meteorology, Commonwealth Scientific and Industrial Research Organisation, Stallergenes Australia, Federal Office of Meteorology and Climatology MeteoSwiss, Switzerland. JMD is an investigator of a National Foundation for Medical Research Innovation grant with co-sponsorship from Abionic Switzerland. JMD is an inventor on patents assigned to QUT. Her institute has received Honorarium payments and travel expenses for education sessions and conference presentations from Stallergenes Australia, Wymedical, and Meda Pharmaceuticals in the last five years. Other authors declare no conflict of interest.

REFERENCES

1. Pawankar R, Canonica GW, Holgate ST, et al, editors. World allergy Organization (WAO) white book on allergy: update 2013. Milwaukee (WI): United States of America; 2013.

2. Sarfaty M, Bloodhart B, Ewart G, et al. American Thoracic Society member survey on climate change and health. Ann Am Thorac Soc 2015;12:274–8.

3. Ozdoganoglu T, Songu M. The burden of allergic rhinitis and asthma. Ther Adv Respir Dis 2012;6:11–23.

4. Pachauri RK, Allen MR, Barros VR, et al. Climate change 2014: synthesis report. Contribution of working groups I, II and III to the fifth assessment report of the intergovernmental panel on climate change. Geneva, Switzerland: IPCC; 2014. p. 151.

5. Sherwood SC. Relative humidity changes in a warmer climate. J Geophys Res 2010;115. https://doi.org/10.1029/2009JD012585.

6. Cleland EE, Chuine I, Menzel A, et al. Shifting plant phenology in response to global change. Trends Ecol Evol 2007;22:357–65.

7. Rafferty NE, Nabity PD. A global test for phylogenetic signal in shifts in flowering time under climate change. J Ecol 2017;105:627–33.

8. Horton RM, Mankin JS, Lesk C, et al. A review of recent advances in research on extreme heat events. Curr Clim Change Rep 2016;2:242–59.

9. Fitter AH, Fitter RS. Rapid changes in flowering time in British plants. Science 2002;296:1689–91.

10. Springer CJ. Ward JK Flowering time and elevated atmospheric CO_2. New Phytol 2007;176:243–55.

11. Ziska LH, Beggs PJ. Anthropogenic climate change and allergen exposure: the role of plant biology. J Allergy Clin Immunol 2012;129:27–32.

12. Goosse H. Reconstructed and simulated temperature asymmetry between continents in both hemispheres over the last centuries. Clim Dyn 2017;48:1483–501.

13. Stouffer RJ, Manabe S, Bryan K. Interhemispheric asymmetry in climate response to a gradual increase of atmospheric CO_2. Nature 1989;342:660–2.

14. Kruger AC, Nxumalo M. Surface temperature trends from homogenized time series in South Africa: 1931–2015. Int J Climat 2017;37:2364–77.

15. Van Nunen S, Dinh NV. Allergy north of the border: parthenium weed allergy. Int Med J 2010;40(Suppl. 4):1–26.

16. Adkins S, Shabbir A. Biology, ecology and management of the invasive parthenium weed (*Parthenium hysterophorus* L.). Pest Man Sci 2014;70:1023–9.

17. Green BJ, Dettmann M, Yli-Panula E, et al. Atmospheric Poaceae pollen frequencies and associations with meteorological parameters in Brisbane, Australia: a 5-year record, 1994–1999. Int J Biomet 2004;48:172–8.

18. Morgan JA, LeCain DR, Pendall E, et al. C_4 grasses prosper as carbon dioxide eliminates desiccation in warmed semi-arid grassland. Nature 2011;476:202–5.

19. García-Mozo H. Poaceae pollen as the leading aeroallergen worldwide: A review. Allergy 2017;72:1849–58.

20. Biganzoli F, Zuloaga F. Análisis de diversidad de la familia Poaceae en la región austral de América del Sur. Rodriguésia 2015;66:337–51.

21. Davies JM. Grass pollen allergens globally: the contribution of subtropical grasses to burden of allergic respiratory diseases. Clin Exp Allergy 2014;44:790–801.

22. Medek DE, Beggs PJ, Erbas B, et al. Regional and seasonal variation in airborne grass pollen levels between cities of Australia and New Zealand. Aerobiologia 2016;32:289–302.

23. Davies JM, Beggs PJ, Medek DE, et al. Trans-disciplinary research in synthesis of grass pollen aerobiology and its importance for respiratory health in Australasia. Sci Total Environ 2015;534:85–96.

24. Seidel DJ, Fu Q, Randel WJ, et al. Widening of the tropical belt in a changing climate. Nat Geosci 2008;1:21–4.
25. Yu Y. Paving the Way for C_4 Evolution: Study of C_3-C_4 Intermediate Species in Grasses. Plant Physiol 2020;182:453.
26. Ramon GD, Barrionuevo LB, Viego V, et al. Sensitization to subtropical grass pollen in patients with seasonal allergic rhinitis from Bahia Blanca, Argentina. WAO J 2019;12:100062.
27. Joubert G. Allergen sensitivities of patients with allergic rhinitis presenting to the ENT Clinic, Universitas Academic Hospital. Curr Allergy Clin Immunol 2006;19:130–2.
28. Kailaivasan TH, Timbrell V, Solley G, et al. Biogeographical variation in specific IgE recognition of temperate and subtropical grass pollen allergens in allergic rhinitis patients. Clin Trans Immunol 2020;9:e1103.
29. Haberle SG, Bowman DMJS, Newnham RM, et al. The macroecology of airborne pollen in Australian and New Zealand urban areas. PLoS One 2014;9:e97925.
30. Australian Institute of Health and Welfare 2019. Allergic rhinitis ('hay fever'). Cat. no. PHE 257. Canberra (Australia): AIHW; 2020. https://www.aihw.gov.au/reports/chronic-respiratory-conditions/allergic-rhinitis-hay-fever. Accessed May 2, 2020.
31. Bousquet P-J, Leynaert B, Neukirch F, et al. Geographical distribution of atopic rhinitis in the European Community Respiratory Health Survey I. Allergy 2008;63:1301–9.
32. Beggs PJ. Climate change and allergy in Australia: an innovative, high-income country, at potential risk. Public Health Res Pract 2018;28:e2841828.
33. Bousquet P-J, Chinn S, Janson C, et al. Geographical variation in the prevalence of positive skin tests to environmental aeroallergens in the European Community Respiratory Health Survey I. Allergy 2007;62:301–9.
34. Davies JM, Dang TD, Voskamp A, et al. Functional immunoglobulin E cross-reactivity between Pas n 1 of Bahia grass pollen and other group 1 grass pollen allergens. Clin Exp Allergy 2011;41:281–91.
35. Hollams EM, Deverell M, Serralha M, et al. Elucidation of asthma phenotypes in atopic teenagers through parallel immunophenotypic and clinical profiling. J Allergy Clin Immunol 2009;124:463–70.
36. Gibbs JEM. Eucalyptus pollen allergy and asthma in children: a cross-sectional study in South-East Queensland, Australia. PLoS ONE 2015;10:e0126506.
37. Bass DJ, Delpech V, Beard J. Late summer and fall (March–May) pollen allergy and respiratory disease in Northern New South Wales, Australia. Ann Allergy Asthma Immunol 2000;85:374–81.
38. Zar HJ, Ehrlich RI, Workman L, et al. The changing prevalence of asthma, allergic rhinitis and atopic eczema in African adolescents from 1995 to 2002. Ped All Immun 2007;18:560–5.
39. Katelaris CH, Burke TV, Byth K. Spatial variability in the pollen count in Sydney, Australia: can one sampling site accurately reflect the pollen count for a region? Ann Allergy Asthma Immunol 2004;93:131–6.
40. Sercombe JK1, Green BJ, Rimmer J, et al. London Plane Tree bioaerosol exposure and allergic sensitization in Sydney, Australia. Ann Allergy Asthma Immunol 2011;107:493–500.
41. de Morton J, Bye J, Pezza A, et al. On the causes of variability in amounts of airborne grass pollen in Melbourne, Australia. Int J Biometeorol 2011;55:613–22.
42. Beggs PJ, Katelaris CH, Medek D, et al. Differences in grass pollen allergen exposure across Australia. Aust N Z J Public Health 2015;39:51–5.

43. Devadas R, Huete AR, Vicendese D, et al. Dynamic ecological observations from satellites inform aerobiology of allergenic grass pollen. Sci Total Environ 2018; 633:441–51.

44. Lynch AJJ, Thackway R, Specht A, et al. Transdisciplinary synthesis for ecosystem science, policy and management: the Australian experience. Sci Total Environ 2015;534:173–84.

45. Lindstrom SJ, Silver JD, Sutherland MF, et al. Thunderstorm asthma outbreak of November 2016: a natural disaster requiring planning. Med J Aust 2017;207: 235–7.

46. Lee J, Kronborg C, O'Hehir RE, et al. Who's at risk of thunderstorm asthma? The ryegrass pollen trifecta and lessons learnt from the Melbourne thunderstorm epidemic. Respir Med 2017;132:146–8.

47. Thien F, Beggs PJ, Csutoros D, et al. The Melbourne epidemic thunderstorm asthma event 2016: an investigation of environmental triggers, effect on health services, and patient risk factors. Lancet Planet Health 2018;2:e255–63.

48. Davies J, Erbas B, Simunovic M, et al. Literature review on thunderstorm asthma and its implications for public health advice. Victorian Department of Health and Human Services; 2017. Available at: https://www2.health.vic.gov.au/public-health/environmental-health/climate-weather-and-public-health/thunderstorm-asthma/response. Accessed October 16, 2020.

49. Beggs PJ, Davies JM, Milic A, et al. Australian Airborne Pollen and Spore Monitoring Network Interim Standard and Protocols. Version 2, 14 September 2018. 77 pp. Available at: https://www.allergy.org.au/images/stories/pospapers/Australian_Pollen_and_Spore_Monitoring_Interim_Standard_and_Protocols_v2_14092018.pdf. Accessed October 16, 2020.

50. Ziska LH, Makra L, Harry SK, et al. Temperature-related changes in airborne allergenic pollen abundance and seasonality across the northern hemisphere: a retrospective data analysis. Lancet Planet Health 2019;3:e124–31.

51. Milic A, Addison-Smith B, Jones PJ, et al. Quality control of pollen identification and quantification exercise for the AusPollen Aerobiology Collaboration Network: a pilot study. Aerobiologia 2020;36:83–7.

52. Berman D. Variations in pollen and fungal air Spora: an analysis of 30 years of monitoring for the clinical assessment of patients in the Western Cape. PhD thesis. University of Cape Town; 2018.

53. Berman D. Climate change and aeroallergens in South Africa. Curr Allergy Clin Immun 2011;24:65–71.

54. Hill TR. Statistical determination of sample size and contemporary pollen counts, Natal Drakensberg, South Africa. Grana 1996;35(2):119–24.

55. Ramón GD, Long A, Barrionuevo LB. Atlas Alergo-palinologico de la República Argentina. Asociacion Argentina de Alergia e Inmunologia Clinica, Moreno 909. Argentina: CABA; 2019. Available at: https://www.alergia.org.ar/index.php/profesionales/conteo-de-polenes. Accessed October 17, 2020.

56. Berman D. Regional-specific pollen and fungal spore allergens in South Africa. Curr Allergy Clin Immunol 2013;26:196.

57. European Committee for Standardization. 2015. Technical Specification: Ambient air - Sampling and analysis of airborne pollen grains and fungal spores for allergy networks - Volumetric Hirst method. Ref. No. CEN/TS 16868:2015.

58. European Standard EN 16868:2019 Ambient air - Sampling and analysis of airborne pollen grains and fungal spores for networks related to allergy - Volumetric Hirst method. Available at: https://www.cen.eu/news/brief-news/pages/en-2019-026.aspx. Accessed October 16, 2020.

59. Galan C, Smith M, Thibaudon M, et al, EAS QC Working Group. Pollen monitoring: minimum requirements and reproducibility of analysis. Aerobiologia 2014;30:385–95.
60. Van Vliet AJ, Overeem A, De Groot RS, et al. The influence of temperature and climate change on the timing of pollen release in the Netherlands. Int J Climatol 2002;22:1757–67.
61. Ziello C, Sparks TH, Estrella N, et al. Changes to airborne pollen counts across Europe. PLoS ONE 2012;7:e34076.
62. Ziska L, Knowlton K, Rogers C, et al. Recent warming by latitude associated with increased length of ragweed pollen season in central North America. Proc Nat Acad Sci U S A 2011;108:4248–51.
63. Miki K, Kawashima S, Clot B, et al. Comparative efficiency of airborne pollen concentration evaluation in two pollen sampler designs related to impaction and changes in internal wind speed. Atmos Env 2019;203:18–27.
64. Frenz DA. Comparing pollen and spore counts collected with the Rotorod Sampler and Burkard spore trap. Ann Allergy Asthma Immunol 1999;83:341–9.
65. Frenz DA. Interpreting atmospheric pollen counts for use in clinical allergy: allergic symptomology. Ann Allergy Asthma Immunol 2001;86:150–8.
66. Addison-Smith E, Wraith D, Davies JM. Standardising pollen monitoring: quantifying confidence intervals for measurements of airborne pollen concentration. Aerobiologia 2020. https://doi.org/10.1007/s10453-020-09656-6.
67. Jato V, Rodríguez-Rajo FJ, Alcázar P, et al. May the definition of pollen season influence aerobiological results? Aerobiologia 2006;22:13.
68. Pfaar O, Bastl K, Berger U, et al. Defining pollen exposure times for clinical trials of allergen immunotherapy for pollen induced rhinoconjunctivitis – an EAACI Position Paper. Allergy 2017;72:713–22.
69. Bastl K, Kmenta M, Berger UE. Defining pollen seasons: background and recommendations. Curr Allergy Asthma Rep 2018;18:73.
70. Galan C, Ariatti A, Bonini M, et al. Recommended terminology for aerobiological studies. Aerobiologia 2017;33:293–5.
71. Cook M, Douglas JA, Mallon D, et al. The economic impact of allergic disease in Australia: not to be sneezed at. Australia. Access Economics Pty Ltd; 2007. for the Australasian Society for Clinical Immunology and Allergy (ASCIA).
72. Rimmer J, Davies J. Hay fever – an underappreciated and chronic disease. Med Today 2015;16:14–24.
73. Ziska LH, Bradley BA, Wallace RD, et al. Climate change, carbon dioxide, and pest biology, managing the future: coffee as a case study. Agronomy 2018;8: 152–7.
74. Campbell B, Al Kouba J, Noor M et al. Tracking temporal changes in pollen diversity by targeted sequencing of the pollen Aerobiome; the Next Stage in aerobiology. 11th International Congress on Aerobiology; Advances in aerobiology for the preservation of human and environmental health: a multidisciplinary approach. Parma Italy September 3-7, 2018.
75. Brennan GL, Potter C, de Vere N, et al. Temperate airborne grass pollen defined by spatio-temporal shifts in community composition. *Nat Ecol* Evol 2019;3:750–4.
76. Oteros J, Pusch G, Weichenmeier I, et al. Automatic and online pollen monitoring. Arch Allergy Immun 2015;167:158–66.
77. Šaulienė I, Šukienė L, Daunys G. Automatic pollen recognition with the Rapid-E particle counter: the first-level procedure, experience and next steps. Atmos Meas Tech 2019;12:3435–52.

78. Sauvageat E, Zeder Y, Auderset K, et al. Real-time pollen monitoring using digital holography. Atmos Meas Tech 2020;13:1539–50.
79. EUMETNET. AutoPollen. Available at: https://www.eumetnet.eu/activities/miscellaneous/current-activities-mi/autopollen/. Accessed February 19, 2020.
80. Ziska LH, Gebhard DE, Frenz DA, et al. Cities as harbingers of climate change: common ragweed, urbanization, and public health. J Allergy Clin Immunol 2003; 111:290–5.
81. Cai W, Wang G, Santoso A, et al. Increased frequency of extreme La Niña events under greenhouse warming. Nat Clim Change 2015;5:132–7.
82. Borchers NA, Palmer AJ, Bowman, et al. Unprecedented smoke-related health burden associated with the 2019–20 bushfires in eastern Australia. Med J Aust 2020. https://doi.org/10.5694/mja2.50545.
83. Gleason JA, Bielory L, Fagliano JA. Associations between ozone, PM2. 5, and four pollen types on emergency department pediatric asthma events during the warm season in New Jersey: a case-crossover study. Environ Res 2014; 132:421–9.
84. Allen JT, Karoly DJ, Walsh KJ. Future Australian severe thunderstorm environments. Part II: The influence of a strongly warming climate on convective environments. J Clim 2014;27:3848–68.
85. Singh MS, Kuang Z, Maloney ED, et al. Increasing potential for intense tropical and subtropical thunderstorms under global warming. Proc Nat Acad Sci U S A 2017;114:11657–62.
86. Klein T, Kukkonen J, Dahl Å, et al. Interactions of physical, chemical, and biological weather calling for an integrated approach to assessment, forecasting, and communication of air quality. Ambio 2012;41:851–64.
87. Watts N, Amann M, Arnell N, et al. The 2019 report of The Lancet Countdown on health and climate change: ensuring that the health of a child born today is not defined by a changing climate. Lancet 2019;394:1836–78.
88. Silver JD, Spriggs K, Haberle SG, et al. Using crowd-sourced allergic rhinitis symptom data to improve grass pollen forecasts and predict individual symptoms. Sci Total Environ 2020;720:137351.
89. Bastl K, Bastl M, Bergmann KC, et al. Translating the burden of pollen allergy into numbers using electronically generated symptom data from the patient's hayfever diary in Austria and Germany: 10-Year Observational Study. J Med Internet Res 2020;22:e16767.
90. Davies JM, Pollen Allergens. In: Nriagu, J. (Ed.), Encyclopedia of environmental health. Elsevier, vol. 5, pp. 300–322. Available at: https://dx.doi.org/10.1016/B978-0-12-409548-9.11537-4 ISBN: 9780444639516, Copyright © 2019 Elsevier B.V. Accessed October 16, 2020.

Allergenic Pollen Season Variations in the Past Two Decades Under Changing Climate in the United States

Divya Seth, MD[a],*, Leonard Bielory, MD[b,c]

KEYWORDS

- Climate change • Pollen • Pollen indices • Allergy

KEY POINTS

- Climate change has contributed to an increase in prevalence of allergic airway diseases.
- Climate factors (increasing temperature and carbon dioxide levels) increase production of pollen, which also exhibit increased allergenicity.
- Climate change has contributing to shift in flowering phenology (trees and ragweed) and pollen initiation, thus causing longer pollen exposure.

INTRODUCTION

Allergic airway diseases (AADs) are common chronic diseases affecting one-third of the population in the United States.[1] Estimated costs of care are approximately $21 billion annually.[2] Among these, allergic rhinoconjunctivitis, allergic sinusitis, and asthma are associated with aeroallergen exposure. The prevalence of these allergic diseases has been increasing over the past 3 decades.[3] This has been related to multiple factors, including obesity, hygiene hypothesis, altered gene-environment interactions, climate change, and pollutants.[4] Overall, there appears to a multifaceted interaction of the various factors that has culminated in the transformations in phenology, production of pollen, distribution of floristic zones, and sensitivity to aeroallergens and may even include the development to new allergens.

Climate change has had and continues to have impact on various allergenic plants. Specific climate factors, including humidity, rising temperatures, and increasing carbon dioxide (CO_2) levels, have resulted in increased production of

[a] Department of Pediatrics, Children's Hospital of Michigan, Central Michigan University, 3950 Beaubien, 4th Floor, Pediatric Specialty Building, Detroit, MI 48201, USA; [b] Center of Environmental Prediction, Rutgers University; [c] Allergy, Immunology, and Ophthalmology, Hackensack Meridian School of Medicine at Seton Hall University, 400 Mountain Avenue, Springfield, NJ 07081, USA
* Corresponding author.
E-mail address: dseth@dmc.org

Immunol Allergy Clin N Am 41 (2021) 17–31
https://doi.org/10.1016/j.iac.2020.09.006
0889-8561/21/© 2020 Elsevier Inc. All rights reserved.

immunology.theclinics.com

pollen, mold, and allergenic plant species for example, toxicondron.[5] In addition to increased quantity, pollen from trees grown under increased temperatures exhibit increased allergenicity.[6] Increasing levels of greenhouse gases (CO_2 and ozone [O_3]) have led to alterations in normal flora (allergen content, geographic distribution, and genetics of plants) and fauna (changes in habitat and allergen content of stinging insects) that provide the basis for increased sensitization and exacerbation of existing AADs (**Fig. 1**). Increased pollen levels in the air increases the efficiency of wind-borne pollination, resulting in dispersion of the pollen over long distances. Over time this will result in increase in aeroallergen burden and an increase in inhalant allergy.[7,8] Climate change is expected to have dual effect on the allergic diseases — on one hand, it affects pollen indices, including the start, duration, and intensity of the pollen season; on the other hand, it affects frequency of AAD, including asthma exacerbations. The presence of allergic sensitization of the nasal and bronchial mucosa also may lead to increased propensity of developing viral respiratory infections, such as coronavirus disease (COVID 19).[9]

Studies have shown climate change (milder winters, warmer air temperatures, and higher CO_2 concentrations) globally is resulting in shifting of plant phenology.[10] Global warming hastens flowering of the plants and early blooming. Compared with the early 1960s, there has been advancement of spring events (flowering of trees) by 6 days and delay of fall season events by 5 days.[11] Prolonged ragweed season in the past 2 decades has been shown to be associated with increase in number of frost-free days and delayed fall frosts.[12] This increases allergic sensitization and increased prevalence of allergic diseases. Patients also experience longer duration as well as increased severity of symptoms.[3] Also, increased outdoor allergen levels results in pollen influx into the house, which results in increased personal exposure. Increased CO_2 levels have been shown to have fertilizing effect on plants.[13] Pollen from ragweed increases 30% to 90% when CO_2 levels double.[14] Similar effect has been seen on other plants including poison ivy.[15]

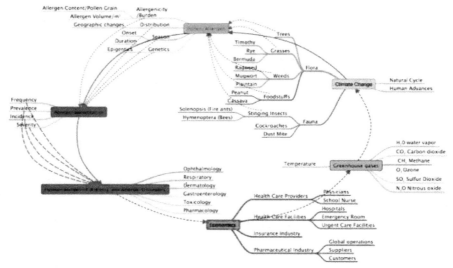

Fig. 1. The cycle of climate and allergic disease. (*From* Bielory L, Lyons K, Goldberg R. Climate change and allergic disease. Curr Allergy Asthma Rep. 2012;12(6): 485-494; with permission.)

AEROBIOLOGY OF NORTH AMERICA

Plants of various species release pollen into the air causing allergy symptoms but only some of these cause significant allergic symptoms (**Table 1**).[16] Epidemiology of allergic diseases is determined by regional pollen distributions, which also is essential for diagnosis and treatment of allergic diseases.

There are 3 distinct plant-based aeroallergen seasons experienced through most of the temperate zones of the United States: tree pollen during spring season, grass pollen in early summer, and weed pollen during end of summer and fall season. Tree and weed pollens can be transported easily over long distances.[16] A variety of weed plants are known to produce very large amount of pollen grains during a season, with ragweed the most commonly sensitized weed in the United States.[16,17] Cutaneous reactivity to ragweed has been reported up to 70% of the US population in the Centers for Disease Control and Prevention National Health and Nutrition Examination Survey studies.[18] Pollen production from trees in various section of the United States, however, may extend beyond spring (*Ulmus* may produce pollen in late summer and early fall; Cupressaceae may produce pollen in fall and winter) and grass pollen may be emitted beyond summers (Poaceae pollen may be released March through November).[16]

Climate change can affect pollen seasons in all of the floristic zones. Floristic zones include the native vegetation found in a particular area and are affected by temperature and mean precipitation. Hardiness zones are characterized by mean annual minimum temperatures. **Fig. 2** depicts difference in hardiness zones from 1990 to 2015.[19]

Table 1
Important pollen in North America

Name	Type of Pollen	Percent	Characteristics
Oak (*Quercus*)	Tree	19.6	Produce heavy pollen load. Found in residential areas, forests, parks
Cyper, juniper, cedar (Cupressaceae)	Tree	19.4	Produce profuse amounts of pollen. Reactions often are severe to Cupressaceae pollen.
Ragweed (*Ambrosia*)	Weed	7.2	Most important cause of rhinitis symptoms in late summer, early fall
Mulberry (*Morus*)	Tree	6.7	Often causes severe reactions
Pine (Pinaceae)	Tree	4.5	Produces large amount of low allergenic pollen
Elm (*Ulmus*)	Tree	4.6	Produces heavy load of allergenic pollen
Ash (Fraxinus)	Tree	3.7	Produces heavy load of allergenic pollen
Birch (*Betula*)	Tree	3.8	Short pollen season.
Grass (Poaceae, Gramineae) (bluegrass, timothy, Bermuda, ryegrass)	Grass	3.7	Poaceae pollen is highly allergenic.
Maple (*Acer*)	Tree	3.7	Most species are allergenic.
Poplar, aspen, cottonwood (*Populus*)	Tree	2.5	Large deciduous trees

Adapted from Lo F, Bitz CM, Battisti DS, et al. Pollen calendars and maps of allergenic pollen in North America. Aerobiologia 2019; 35(4): 613–633; with permission.

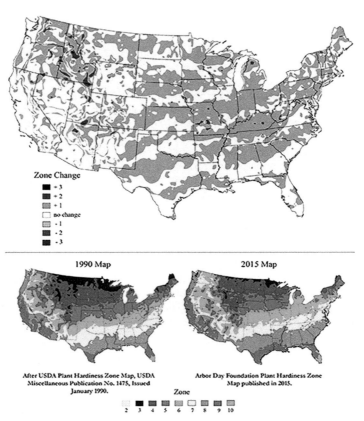

Fig. 2. Differences between 1990 US Department of Agriculture hardiness zones and 2015 Arborday.org hardiness zones. (*From* Differences between 1990 USDA Hardiness Zones and 2015 Arborday.org Hardiness Zones. Arbor Day Foundation. 2015 Available at: https://www.arborday.org/media/map_change.cfm With permission.)

Migration of these zones has happened due to global warming, thereby affecting the type of flora in a given area. Within the United States, there has been 2-zone shift in some areas in the past 2 decades. Over time, there has been a change in distribution of trees. Boreal trees (fir, larch, and alder) have shifted south with cooling, while replaced by oak and white pine (northward shift) with subsequent warming.[20] Lo and colleagues[16] conducted a study to generate data on pollen distribution in the United States and Canada. The investigators used data from 31 National Allergy Bureau (NAB) pollen stations from 2003 to 2017 to develop pollen calendars for specific pollen taxa. It was noted that in most areas, a majority of the total pollen is contributed by only a small number of taxa. For tree and grass pollen season, start date strongly correlates with latitude, which in turn correlates with temperature and length of the day. Earlier start date was noted for lower latitudes. Also, earlier start date correlated with longer pollen season duration.[16]

Various environmental factors contribute to pollen allergy, such as climate and local plantations.[21] Pollen concentrations in a given area correlate with the local weather conditions and vegetation and usually reflect pollen emissions locally,[22] although sometimes they might be transported to farther places.[23]

Pollen calendars are created using daily average pollen concentrations. They help to determine distribution, timing, and concentration of different pollen at a particular location. This allows physicians and patients to identify their allergen triggers and initiate appropriate testing and treatment.[24]

POLLEN SEASON INDICES

Pollen season indices (annual pollen integral [APIn], duration of the pollen season, and start and end dates) are used to describe prominent features of the main pollen season. APIn is defined as the integral of the pollen concentration for a particular taxon measured daily over the pollen year. A pollen year is a year that includes 1 full pollen season, starting when the plant is still dormant. Start date of the pollen season usually is considered when the integral of pollen concentration approaches 50 pollen grains/m^3 during a pollen year. In cases of plants with high APIn (>2000 pollen grain/m^3), end date of the pollen season is defined as the date when the integral of pollen concentration up to the end of the pollen year is less than 50 pollen grain/m^3. In cases of plants with APIn less 2000 pollen grain/m^3, the end date threshold is the date when accumulated pollen concentration approaches 97.5% mean APIn. Most sensitive patients tend to experience symptoms even at low airborne pollen concentrations (50 pollen grains/m^3). This could be related to priming effect of allergens, wherein daily exposure to the allergen results in increased allergic response.[25]

Pollen sensitization occurs when a genetically predisposed individual is exposed to their individual threshold. This varies with geographic location, CO_2 and O_3 levels, climate variations, and air pollution. Pollen levels increase during warm and dry days whereases levels fall during cool and moist days. In recent decades, ragweed pollen season has increased in North America and is related to latitude and linked to warming temperatures in those regions.[12] Over a period of 20 years, from the 1990s to 2010, daily average airborne allergen has increased by 46%.[26] Elevated CO_2 levels have been shown to have increased ragweed pollen production.[27] Additional factors that have an impact on allergenic pollen production include pollution and diesel exhaust.[28,29]

MODELS FOR POLLEN DISPERSAL

AADs comprise a complex medical problem that often is triggered by air pollutants and bioaerosols, but, due to the inability to obtain precise information regarding spatial distribution of bioaerosol emissions, it is difficult to predict their combined effect. Currently, however, there are no standardized methods across the United States that allow estimation of such emissions. Various numerical models have been developed to assess the effect of climate change on pollen emission and transport and the impact on AADs. These models are based on phenological observations or use meteorologic principles.

Pollen Emissions Module

The pollen emissions module provides estimate of pollen particle emissions from common allergenic trees and plants in the United States based on biogenic gas emissions used in the Biogenic Emission Inventory System. Several factors influence pollen emission that include humidity, temperature, speed of wind, and total growing degree days. The Intergovernmental Panel on Climate Change (IPCC) concluded that milder temperatures affect pollen production resulting in early release as well as increased allergenicity.[30] Various remote sensing sources and local surveys were used to develop a spatiotemporal vegetation map, which was coupled with the mesoscale meteorologic model to develop emission rates of various pollens.[31] Strong correlations were noticed between predicted pollen emissions and measured pollen counts across wide geographic region using this approach.

Atmospheric Pollen Transport Module

Different models have been developed for analysis of transport of pollen and transformation of other air pollutants (**Table 2**).[32] Among these, models commonly used in the United States include (1) the Hybrid Single-Particle Lagrangian Integrated Trajectory (HYSPLIT) model and (2) the modified version of US Environmental Protection Agency Community Multiscale Air Quality (CMAQ) model. The CMAQ model offers advantage of being more flexible. The CMAQ model includes 3 different models—meteorologic model, emission model, and air transport model. The meteorologic model represents weather conditions; the emission model represents emissions from man-made as well as natural sources; and the air transport model is used to predict air pollutants transmission based on atmospheric conditions. The CMAQ provides prompt and accurate information regarding O_3, particulate material, toxics, and acid deposition. The CMAQ pollen model uses a single model simulation to predict transport of multiple air pollutants and pollens.

The HYSPLIT model commonly is used to compute atmospheric transport and dispersion of allergens and pollutants. It has been used in simulations models describing transport, chemical transformation, and deposition of bioaerosols and hazardous materials, including radioactive material, wildfire smoke, and volcanic emissions. It often is used for back trajectory analysis, which involves establishing source-receptor relationship to determine origin of these particles. In general, CMAQ estimated profiles correspond with the pollen transport trajectories as estimated by HYSPLIT.[32]

Table 2 Various models developed for large-scale emissions and long-range transport of pollen			
Model for Pollen Transport	Model for Pollen Emission	Species of Plant	Location and Year of the Study
CMAQ model	Meteorologic parameterization	Birch and ragweed	USA (2010)
Aerosols and reactive trace gas (ART) model	Meteorologic parameterization	Birch	Switzerland (2008)
Mesoscale atmospheric meteorology (METRAS) model	Meteorologic parameterization	Oak	Germany (2006)
System for Integrated Modeling of Atmospheric Composition (SILAM)	Phenological observations	Birch	Finland (2006)
HYSPLIT model	Uniform diurnal profile	Oak	USA (2005)
DRAIS chemistry transport model (CTM)	Meteorologic parameterization	Hazel, alder	Germany (2004)
Gaussian model	Meteorologic parameterization	Cedar	Japan(1999)

EFFECT OF CLIMATE CHANGE ON TREE POLLEN

In a study that was conducted to examine the effect of climate change on spatiotemporal patterns of *Betula* (birch) and *Quercus* (oak) tree pollen, data were collected from 6 NAB stations from 1994 to 2011 in order to assess the effect of climate change on trends of annual pollen production (AP), season start, and season length.[33] Comparing data from 1994 to 2000 to 2001 to 2010, birch and oak trees began to pollinate 1 week to 2 weeks earlier during 2000 to 2010. The annual mean pollen concentrations and the daily peak values (PVs) increased at most of the stations for birch and oak trees. Season length for birch was noted to be shorter whereas season lengths for oak varied according to the location.[33]

The growing degree hour model has been used for developing spatiotemporal profiles of pollen emissions and to produce simulated data on future start dates and season lengths for birch and oak tree pollen (year 2050). Simulation results indicated that responses of birch and oak pollen seasons to climate change are projected to vary for different regions based on regional climate variations. As an example, the birch pollen season in 2050 in the Northeastern United States is projected to start earlier and last longer, and in the Northwestern United States, it is projected to start later and end sooner; whereas the oak pollen season in 2050 in Northeastern United States is projected to be longer and, in the Northwestern United States, the season is expected to start earlier. Earlier start dates and longer pollen seasons for both birch and oak pollen in Northeastern United States are linked to increasing temperatures and regional warming.[33]

Bayesian models were used by Zhang and colleagues[34] to study the effect of multiple climate factors on different pollen indices (AP, PV, start date, and peak date) of birch (*Betula*) tree. The model used variable selection-parameterization-evaluation-prediction factors.

The model was developed to assess the impact of climate change related to anthropogenic activities on future pollen indices. It was based on 3 IPCC scenarios (based on economic, demographic, and technological factors): (1) A2—economic development, (2) A1B—economic growth with balanced emphasis on energy sources (A1B), and (3) B1—globally and environmentally oriented development. Each scenario was associated with different projections of CO_2 concentrations (853 parts per million [ppm], 709 ppm, and 533 ppm) and temperature (17.7°C, 17.0°C, and 16.1°C) in 2100. Spatiotemporal emission profiles were developed for birch tree pollen for the Northeastern United States for the years 2002 and 2040 by incorporating predicted pollen integral into the emission model. Among different climate factors, mean spring temperature, annual mean (CO_2) and pollen counts of the prior year had significant effect on the pollen indices. The investigators used the output of these models to formulate birch pollen emissions for future years (from 2020 to 2100), as shown in **Table 3**.

The start and peak dates of birch pollen season are expected to occur 2 weeks to 4 weeks earlier than usual. Climate change, thus, is expected to have significant effects in pollen production, timing, and intensity and subsequently will have a significant impact on patients that suffer from AAD.[34] Pollen release from trees including birch has been earlier and more pronounced across North America.[35] In New England, pollen as well as mold spore counts were highest during a warmer, wetter El Niño year compared with other years.[36] In the San Francisco Bay area, California, pollen counts for oak tree were strongly associated with total rainfall during the preceding year.[37] Over the years, there has been a significant increase in seasonal pollen levels of *Juniperus*, *Quercus*, *Carya*, and *Betula* spp. Certain trees (*Juniperus*, *Ulmus*, and *Morus*) have been having early start dates during pollen season. This was significantly related

Table 3

Comparison of mean pollen counts and related indicators of annual pollen production, peak pollen count values, pollen release start date, and peak pollen count date between 2020 and 2100 starting with the base year 2000

Pollen Index	Scenario	2000	2020	2040	2060	2080	2100
AP (pollen.m^{-3})	B1	8455	11,413 (1.3)	18,286 (2.2)	23,872 (2.8)	26,913 (3.2)	27,621 (3.3)
	A2	8455	12,019 (1.4)	21,047 (2.5)	33,005 (3.9)	47,778 (5.7)	67,831 (8.0)
	A1B	8455	12.673 (1.5)	21,735 (2.6)	31,950 (3.8)	41,518 (4.9)	49,889 (5.9)
PV (pollen.m^{-3})	B1	1684	1844 (1.1)	3121 (1.9)	4187 (2.5)	4768 (3.2)	4918 (3.3)
	A2	1684	1951 (1.2)	3622 (2.2)	5851 (3.5)	8601 (5.1)	12,334 (7.3)
	A1B	1684	2067 (1.2)	3758 (2.2)	5671 (3.4)	7468 (4.4)	9056 (5.4)
Start date (days from January 1)	B1	105	86 (−19)	86 (−19)	85 (−20)	84 (−21)	84 (−21)
	A2	105	86 (−19)	86 (−19)	84 (−21)	83 (−22)	81 (−24)
	A1B	105	86 (−19)	86 (−19)	84 (−21)	83 (−22)	83 (−22)
Peak date (days from January 1)	B1	122	99 (−23)	99 (−23)	98 (−24)	98 (−24)	97 (−25)
	A2	122	99 (−23)	99 (−23)	98 (−24)	97 (−25)	96 (−26)
	A1B	122	99 (−23)	98 (−24)	98 (−24)	97 (−25)	96 (−26)

The ratio to or differences from base year are in parentheses. The model has predicted a dramatic increase in AP (1.3–8.0×) and PVs (1.1–7.3×) of birch pollen. For 2040, AP and PV for 3 scenario A2/A1B/B1 increase to 21,047 (2.4×)/18,286 (2.1×) and 3622 (2.3×)/3758 (2.3×)/3121 (1.9×), respectively. For 2100, AP and PV for A2/A1B/B1 increase to 67,831 (7.6×)/49,889 (5.6×)/27,621 (3.1×) and 12,334 (7.7×)/9056 (5.6×)/4918 (3.1×).

From Zhang Y, Isukapalli S, Bielory L, et al. Bayesian Analysis of Climate Change Effects on Observed and Projected Airborne Levels of Birch Pollen. Atmos Environ. 2013; 68: 64–73 with permission.

to warmer temperatures increasingly seen during winters.[14] A significant increase has been seen in *Juniperus* spp pollen counts in Oklahoma due to encroachment of *Juniperus* spp trees into the native grasslands along with earlier start dates for tree pollen season. The rise in pollen counts of Cupressaceous and *Ulmus* spp correlates with daily temperatures. On the other hand, pollen levels were negatively associated with daily precipitation, because rain washes away the pollen particles.[38] Preseason weather parameters, including temperature and precipitation, also showed significant correlations with pollen parameters. Preseason temperature has been shown essential for maturation and release of pollen from spring-pollinating tree species. This is related to the accumulated temperature above the threshold. As a result, warmer winters are associated with earlier pollen season start dates.[39]

EFFECT ON RAGWEED

The duration of the ragweed (*Ambrosia* spp) pollen season has been increasing in past few years.[12] Increasing duration of ragweed pollen season in North America has been correlated to latitude and thus warming temperatures. The increase in surface temperature has not been uniform all over, rather has been more toward the poles or with increase in altitude.[40] Since 1995, the ragweed pollen season has been longer by 13 days to 27 days at latitudes above 44°N. Ziska and colleagues[12] collected and analyzed data pertaining to ragweed pollen as collected by NAB in in the United States and Aerobiology Research Laboratories in Canada. The aim was to analyze the effect of latitude on the ragweed pollen production in regards to frost-free days as surrogate for temperatures changes related to climate change. The data were collected from 8 NAB locations from latitude of 30.63°N (Austin, Texas) to 46.88°N (Fargo, North Dakota) and 2 locations in Canada from latitude 50.1°N (Winnipeg, Manitoba) to 52.1°N (Saskatoon, Saskatchewan) over a duration of 15 years (**Fig. 3**). The data obtained were statistically analyzed for each location. The investigators noted that the length of the duration of ragweed season was significantly associated with latitude.[12] The investigators then analyzed data for each location. They compared duration of ragweed season against seasonal variations in temperature for each location. They

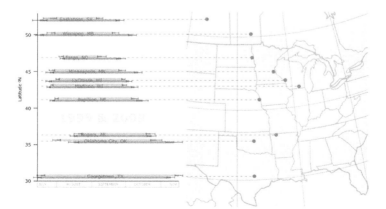

Fig. 3. NAB locations in the United States and Canada used for data collection. (*From* Ziska L, Knowlton K, Rogers C, et al. Recent warming by latitude associated with increased length of ragweed pollen season in central North America. PNAS 2011;108(10): 4248-5; with permission.)

noticed that over the past 15 years, increase in the duration of ragweed season was associated with an increase in number of frost-free days as well as delayed onset of fall frosts (**Fig. 4**), which in turn was noted to have a clear correlation with latitude of each location. There was no correlation between latitude and other weather phenomenon, such as precipitation.[12] In another study, it was determined that same-day total precipitation significantly affects ragweed pollen levels. Changes in daily pollen levels were noted to be inversely related to total precipitation. Rainfall tends to wash away pollen particle and also prevents further dehiscence of the pollen particle.[41]

Ziska and colleagues[21] conducted a study to assess the impact of climate change on ragweed pollen production using a temperature-CO_2 gradient between urban and rural areas to assess the impact for year 2000 and 2001. Average daily CO_2 concentration and air temperature in an urban area were 30% to 31% and 3.4°F to 3.6°F, respectively, more than the rural area. They noticed that the higher temperature and CO_2 concentration in the urban area led to faster growth of ragweed (*Alternaria artemisiifolia*) and earlier and increased pollen production and produced large amounts of above-ground biomass compared with rural areas.[21] In Tulsa, total *Ambrosia* spp pollen levels decreased significantly from 1987 to 2006.[42] Warmer temperatures during August were shown to be a contributing factor, in addition to urbanization. Wan and colleagues showed, however, that warmer temperatures increased *A psilostachya*

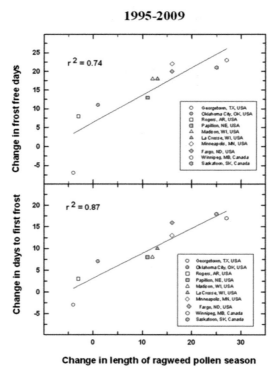

Fig. 4. Change in the length (days) of ragweed pollen season from 1995 to 2009 as a function of frost-free days and delays in the time of first frost during the fall, as a function of latitude. (*From* Ziska L, Knowlton K, Rogers C, et al. Recent warming by latitude associated with increased length of ragweed pollen season in central North America. PNAS 2011;108(10): 4248-5; with permission.)

pollen counts.[43] A psilostachya is perennial wehreas A artemisiifolia is annual. Thus, there might be a difference in the response of perennial versus annual ragweed spp. Response of ragweed pollen season to climate change was analyzed in 9 climate regions across the United States. Spatiotemporal distributions of ragweed pollen were simulated during 2001 to 2004 and 2047 to 2050 to study the effect of climate change on ragweed pollen season timing and levels in the different climate region. As shown in **Table 4**, the pollen season length was short in all climate regions across the United States. The mean hourly concentration decreased in 6 of the 9 regions. The maximum hourly concentration increased in 5 of the 9 regions, with the effect being most pronounced in the East North Central region (34.7% increase). The pollen season was predicted to start late in 7 of the 9 regions.[44]

Zhang and colleagues[25] conducted a study to analyze the effect of climate change on the pollen season for trees (birch and oak), grasses (Poaceae), and weeds (ragweed and mugwort weed). The investigators described the spatiotemporal patterns of changes in the levels and timing of pollen belonging to multiple taxa that are exposed to different climate across the United States. They obtained daily pollen counts from all 50 NAB stations across the United States from 1994 to 2010, expressed as pollen grains per cubic meter.[26] Analysis of the data showed that of the 50 stations, early start dates were seen at a majority of the stations for all different taxa. Season length was shorter for birch and oak stations but longer for ragweed, mugwort, and grass at more than half of the stations. Also, PV and AP showed increasing trend for spring-flowering taxa (birch, oak, and grass) at 62% stations whereas for summer flowering (ragweed and mugwort) taxa, a decreasing trend was more common.[26] Pollen indices during the period 2000 to 2010 were compared with those of 1990s. Pollen season was noted to start earlier by an average of 3 days for all different taxa (trees, grasses, and weeds) during 2001 to 2010 in most of the climate regions. Also, pollen levels increased to a

Table 4
Regional average and SD of the changes in mean and maximum hourly concentrations, start date, season length, and exceedance hours for ragweed (*Ambrosia*) pollen

Regions	Mean Hourly (%)	Maximum Hourly (%)	Start Date (Days) − = Earlier, + = Later	Season Length (Days)	Exceedance Hours (>30 Grains/m³) (%)
NW	−8.7 ±26.2	−10.6 ±41	1.2 ±1.3	−1.1 ±1	−5.5 ±25.7
WNC	0.8 ±22.2	0.9 ±45.3	1.7 ±1	−2 ±0.9	3.5 ±47.1
ENC	−3.4 ±16.5	34.7 ±98.3	1.8 ±1.2	−3.7 ±0.9	−3 ±17.3
NE	−9.3 ±43.8	−19.3 ±74.7	−0.9 ±1.5	−0.9 ±0.8	−6.2 ±111.8
W	−36.4 ±19.1	−30.5 ±23	0.5 ±1.2	−0.3 ±1	−11 ±25.7
C	2 ±30.7	13.8 ±91	1 ±1.1	−3.8 ±1	4.1 ±81.1
SW	15.2 ±39.7	13.1 ±78	0.1 ±1.1	−0.7 ±0.8	6.2 ±42.7
SE	−9.6 ±34.3	−23 ±59.6	−1.1 ±0.7	−0.2 ±0.5	−8.6 ±46.2
S	−1.8 ±30.3	17.7 ±128.7	0.3 ±1	−1.4 ±0.7	−2.8 ±28.9

Abbreviations: C, Central; ENC, East North Central; NE, Northeast; NW, Northwest; S, South; SE, Southeast; SW, Southwest; W, West; WNC, West North Central.

These changes were calculated using the simulation data between periods of 2001 to 2004 and 2047 to 2050 in 9 climate regions across the United States (mean ±SD).

From Zhang Y. Climate Change and Airborne Allergens[dissertation]. New Brunswick, Rutgers. 2015. Available at: https://rucore.libraries.rutgers.edu/rutgers-lib/46460/.

great extent compared with 1990s. The average peak pollen count and annual airborne pollen production increased by 42.4% and 46.0%, respectively. Length of the pollen season, however, was noted to vary: in the northeastern regions, the pollen season lasted longer whereas in southern region, the pollen season was shorter than in 1990s. Pollen seasons were shorter for spring flowering plants by 3.1 days to 4.8 days and longer for summer flowering taxa (ragweed and mugwort) by 1.3 days to 10 days.[26] The investigators also noticed that these changes in pollen levels and season timing were related to latitude. At higher latitudes, the pollen seasons were noted to start earlier and also the length of the pollen season increased. Higher latitudes also experienced larger changes in average AP but only smaller changes in average peak pollen levels.[26] Thus, recent climate change, especially enhanced warming and precipitation at higher latitudes, has resulted in longer and more intense pollen exposure, thereby increasing the prevalence of AAD. These climate changes have resulted in a similar shift in plants and animal distribution.[45] Changes in precipitation have resulted in dual effects. Increased precipitation washes away airborne pollen resulting in decreased peak airborne pollen levels. Larger increase in precipitation, however, seen at higher latitudes, has been more favorable for growth of plants, thereby resulting in higher levels of pollen. This dual effect is seen to be more prominent on the higher latitudes, which, if it continues, can lead to increased prevalence of AADs and increased morbidity related to early start dates and increased exposure to airborne pollens.

Climate change and higher CO_2 concentrations have resulted in increased spore production of *Alternaria alternata* (common allergenic mold), contributing to increased occurrence of asthma and other allergic diseases.[46] A study conducted in Denver, Colorado, analyzed the relationship between certain climate factors (humidity, temperature, sunshine, and wind) and observed tree, grass, and weed pollen levels. Weed pollen levels were more affected by temperature and were noted to be low after an early fall frost in Denver. On the other hand, tree pollen and grass pollen were affected more by precipitation. Association between climate factors and pollen level, however, was not consistent and varied from year to year.[47] Experimental warming has been shown to induce flowering earlier in plants that flower in spring and early summer whereas delayed flowering was seen in late summer and fall flowering plants. *Ambrosia* spp exhibited delayed flowering related to a prolonged bud stage. There was a significant change in flowering time of 2 summer flowering grasses—advanced flowering in *Panicum* spp (17 days early) whereas delayed flowering in *Andropogon* spp (10 days later).[48] Climate change can have a significant impact on AADs through exposure to new allergens or higher concentrations of indigenous aeroallergens. Both pollen and dust can be dispersed over long distances. In Tulsa, Oklahoma, *Juniperus ashei* pollen gets dispersed over long distances and contributes to increased allergic symptoms in the area.[49]

SUMMARY

Climate change, over the years, has contributed significantly to an increase in prevalence of AADs. Effect of climate change also has been seen on plant distribution as seen in widespread expansion of *Juniperus* spp in central and the southwest United States. Future research needs to focus on collecting long-term integrated data series on different allergenic pollen species. The results also can be extrapolated to document future changes in pollen production and distribution with assessment models that would integrate socioeconomic factors, climate factors, and technological changes. Research can help develop more sustainable and effective measures for control of aeroallergens.

CLINICS CARE POINTS

- Climate change globally has contributed to an increase in prevalence and severity of AADs related to altered pollen production as well as timing and duration of pollen season.
- Complex interaction between increasing pollen levels and air pollutants can increase the burden of asthma and other allergic diseases further.
- Anthropogenic activities have resulted in increased production of greenhouse gases (CO_2 and O_3), which in turn have led to global warming and climate change.
- Climate change (increasing temperatures and CO_2) have contributed to increased allergenicity of plants.
- Climate change also has affected the distribution and type of trees and other vegetation over recent years in a geographic area.

DISCLOSURE

The authors have nothing to disclose.

REFERENCES

1. Bielory L, Lyons K, Goldberg R. Climate change and allergic disease. Curr Allergy Asthma Rep 2012;12:485–94.
2. Centers for Disease Control and Prevention. Allergies and Hayfever 2005. Available at: www.cdc.gov/nchs/fastabs/allergies.htm. Accessed February 3, 2011.
3. United States Environmental Protection Agency. A review of the impact of climate variability and change in aeroallergens and their associated effects (final report). Washington, DC: US EPA; 2008. EPA/600/R-06/164F.
4. Beggs PJ, Bambrick HJ. Is the global rise of asthma an early impact of anthropogenic climate change? Environ Health Perspect 2005;113(8):915–9.
5. Bielory L, Deener A. Seasonal variation in the effects of major indoor and outdoor environmental variables on asthma. J Asthma 1998;35(1):7–48.
6. Ahlholm JU, Helander ML, Savolainen J. Genetic and environmental factors affecting the allergenicity of birch (Betula pubescens ssp. czerepanovii [Orl.] Hamet-ahti) pollen. Clin Exp Allergy 1998;28(11):1384–8.
7. Singh K, Axelrod S, Bielory L. The epidemiology of ocular and nasal allergy in the United States, 1988-1994. J Allergy Clin Immunol 2010;126(4):778–83.e6.
8. Meng Q, Nagarajan S, Son Y, et al. Asthma, oculonasal symptoms, and skin test sensitivity across National Health and Nutrition Examination Surveys. Ann Allergy Asthma Immunol 2016;116:118–25.
9. Gilles S, Blume C, Wimmer M, et al. Pollen exposure weakens innate defense against respiratory viruses. Allergy 2020;75:576–87.
10. Cleland EE, Chuine I, Menzel A, et al. Shifting plant phenology in response to global change. Trends Ecol Evol 2007;22:357–65.
11. Menzel A. Trends in phenological phases in Europe between 1951 and 1996. Int J Biometeorol 2000;44(2):76–81.
12. Ziska L, Knowlton K, Rogers C, et al. Recent warming by latitude associated with increased length of ragweed pollen season in central North America. Proc Natl Acad Sci U S A 2011;108:4248–51.

13. Ziska L, Bunce J, Goins E. Characterization of an urban-rural CO2/temperature gradient and associated changes in initial plant productivity during secondary succession. Oecologia 2004;139:454–8.
14. Levetin E. Effects of climate change on airborne pollen. J Allergy Clin Immunol 2001;107:S172.
15. Mohan JE, Ziska LH, Schlesinger WH, et al. Biomass and toxicity responses of poison ivy (Toxicodendron radicans) to elevated atmospheric CO2. Proc Natl Acad Sci U S A 2006;103:9086–9.
16. Lo F, Bitz CM, Battisti DS, et al. Pollen calendars and maps of allergenic pollen in North America. Aerobiologia 2019;35:613–33.
17. Wodehouse RP. Hayfever plants. 2nd edition. New York): Hafner; 1971.
18. Gergen PJ, Turkeltaub PC, Kovar MG. The prevalence of allergic skin test reactivity to eight common aeroallergens in the U.S. population: results from the second National Health and Nutrition Examination Survey. J Allergy Clin Immunol 1987;80:669–79.
19. Arbor Day Foundation. Zone changes: USDA plant hardiness zones. 2006. Available at: www.arborday.org/media/mapchanges.cfm. Accessed February 3, 2011.
20. Beggs PJ. Environmental allergens: from asthma to hay fever and beyond. Curr Clim Change Rep 2015;1(3):176–84.
21. Ziska LH, Gebhar DE, Frenz DA, et al. Cities as harbingers of climate change: common ragweed, urbanization, and public health. J Allergy Clin Immunol 2003;111(2):290–5.
22. Keynan N, Waisel Y, Shomer-Ilan A, et al. Annual variations of air-borne pollen in the Coastal Plain of Israel. Grana 1991;30(2):477–80.
23. Sofiev M, Siljamo P, Ranta H, et al. Towards numerical forecasting of long-range air transport of birch pollen: theoretical considerations and a feasibility study. Int J Biometeorol 2006;50:392–402.
24. Katotomichelakis M, Nikolaidis C, Makris M, et al. The clinical significance of the pollen calendar of the Western Thrace/northeast Greece region in allergic rhinitis. Int Forum Allergy Rhinol 2015;5(12):1156–63.
25. Prince A, Norris MR, Bielory L. Seasonal ocular allergy and pollen counts. Curr Opin Allergy Clin Immunol 2008;18(5):387–92.
26. Zhang Y, Bielory L, Mi Z, et al. Allergenic pollen season variations in the past two decades under changing climate in the United States. Glob Chang Biol 2015;21:1581–9.
27. Ziska L, Caulfield F. Rising carbon dioxide and pollen production of common ragweed, a known allergy-inducing species: implications for public health. Aust J Plant Physiol 2000;27:893–8.
28. D'Amato G, Cecchi L, Bonini S, et al. Allergenic pollen and pollen allergy in Europe. Allergy 2007;62:976–90.
29. Knox RB, Suphioglu C, Taylor P, et al. Major grass pollen allergen Lol p 1 binds to diesel exhaust particles: implications for asthma and air pollution. Clin Exp Allergy 1997;27:246–51.
30. IPCC. Climate change 2007: the physical science basis. In: Solomon S, Qin D, Manning M, et al, editors. Contribution of Working Group I to the Fourth assessment Report of the Intergovernmental Panel on climate change. New York: Cambridge University Press; 2007. p. 996.
31. Grell GA, Dudhia J, Stauffer DR. A Description of the fifth-Generation Penn state/NCAR Mesoscale model (MM5). Boulder (CO): National Center for Atmospheric Research; 1996. p. 88. Report No.: NCAR Technical Note NCAR/TN–398+STR.

32. Efstathiou C, Isukapalli S, Georgopoulos P. A mechanistic modeling system for estimating large scale emissions and transport of pollen and co-allergens. Atmos Environ 2011;45(13):2260–76.
33. Zhang Y, Bielory L, Georgopoulos PG. Climate change effect on Betula (birch) and Quercus (oak) pollen seasons in the United States. Int J Biometeorol 2014; 58(5):909–19.
34. Zhang Y, Isukapalli S, Bielory L, et al. Bayesian analysis of climate change effects on observed and projected airborne levels of birch pollen. Atmos Environ 2013; 68:64–73.
35. Levetin E, Van de Water P. Changing pollen types/concentrations/distribution in the United States: fact or fiction? Curr Allergy Asthma Rep 2008;8:418–24.
36. Freye HB, King J, Litwin CM. Variations of pollen and mold concentrations in 1998 during the strong El Nino event of 1997–1998 and their impact on clinical exacerbations of allergic rhinitis, asthma, and sinusitis. Allergy Asthma Proc 2001; 22:239–47.
37. Weber RW. Meteorologic variables in aerobiology. Immunol Allergy Clin North Am 2003;23(3):411–22.
38. Shea KM, Truckner RT, Weber RW, et al. Climate change and allergic disease. J Allergy Clin Immunol 2008;122:443–53.
39. Peteet D. Sensitivity and rapidity of vegetational response to abrupt climate change. Proc Natl Acad Sci U S A 2000;97:1359–61.
40. Dvorin DJ, Lee JJ, Belecanech GA, et al. A comparative, volumetric survey of airborne pollen in Philadelphia, Pennsylvania (1991-1997) and Cherry Hill, New Jersey (1995-1997). Ann Allergy Asthma Immunol 2001;87:394–404.
41. Solomon WR. Aerobiology of pollinosis. J Allergy Clin Immunol 1984;74:449–61.
42. Levetin E, Avery J. Long term trends in airborne ragweed pollen in Tulsa, Oklahoma: 1987 to 2006. J Allergy Clin Immunol 2008;121(2):S21.
43. Wan S, Yuan T, Bowdish S, et al. Response of an allergenic species, Ambrosia psilostachya (Asteraceae), to experimental warming and clipping: implications for public health. Am J Bot 2002;89(11):1843–6.
44. Zhang Y. Climate change and airborne allergens[dissertation] new Brunswick, Rutgers. The State University of New Jersey; 2015.
45. Inouye DW, Barr B, Armitage KB, et al. Climate change is affecting altitudinal migrants and hibernating species. Proc Natl Acad Sci U S A 2000;97:1630–3.
46. Wolf J, O'Neill NR, Rogers CA, et al. Elevated atmospheric carbon dioxide concentrations amplify alternaria alternata sporulation and total antigen production. Environ Health Perspect 2010;118:1223–8.
47. Glassheim JW, Ledoux RA, Vaughan TR, et al. Analysis of Meteorologic Variables and Seasonal Aeroallergen Pollen Counts in Denver, Colorado. Ann Allergy Asthma Immunol 1995;75(2):149–56.
48. Sherry RA, Zhou X, Gu S, et al. Divergence of reproductive phenology under climate warming. Proc Natl Acad Sci U S A 2007;104(1):198–202.
49. Van de Water PK, Keever T, Main C, et al. An assessment of predictive forecasting of Juniperus ashei pollen movement in the Southern Great Plains, USA. Int J Biometeorol 2003;48(2):74–82.

Climate Change and Pollen Allergy in India and South Asia

Anand Bahadur Singh, PhD[a],*, Chandni Mathur, PhD[a,b]

KEYWORDS

- Climate change • Pollen allergy • Pollinosis • Increased CO_2 • Phenology
- Global warming • India • Southeast Asia

KEY POINTS

- Anthropogenic emissions continue to increase in one form or other.
- Health impacts are increasing with de novo symptoms, such as impaired immune tolerance.
- Massive movement/momentum is needed to reduce emissions of greenhouse gases such as CO_2 emissions across the globe.

The defining concern and challenge for medical science worldwide is the continuously increasing burden of ill-health, low quality of life, and socioeconomic inequality arising because of noncommunicable diseases (NCDs). The limited medical facilities and low economic status are unavoidable factors, especially for the urban poor in developing countries. NCDs principally include cardiovascular diseases, diabetes, cancer, and chronic respiratory diseases. The increasing incidence of respiratory diseases, including allergic rhinitis and asthma, has been attributed to air pollution, climate change, and urbanization affecting both humans and the biosphere.[1] Increasing epidemiology-based studies are stressing new cases of respiratory disorders such as rhinitis and asthma, especially among vulnerable groups such as children and older adults, arising because of climate change, the high rate of global warming, and air pollution.[2] Climate change threatens the last 50 years of gains made in public health.[3]

Allergic diseases are a result of the intricate interaction of genetic makeup and environmental factors. The timing of exposure to the allergenic precursors as sensitizing agents is a determining factor in the long-term incidence and prevalence of allergic diseases.

a CSIR-Institute of Genomics & Integrative Biology, University Campus, Delhi, India; b B-702 Amrapali Apartment, Sector-3 Vaishali, Ghaziabad 201010, Uttar Pradesh, India
* Corresponding author. A-4 Shanti Apartments, Sector-13 Rohini, Delhi 110085, India,
E-mail address: singha49@hotmail.com

Immunol Allergy Clin N Am 41 (2021) 33–52
https://doi.org/10.1016/j.iac.2020.09.007
0889-8561/21/© 2020 Elsevier Inc. All rights reserved.
immunology.theclinics.com

For respiratory disorders, broadly the risk factors are occupational agents, indoor pollution from cooking fuel and tobacco smoke, and environmental exposure to air pollutants from traffic and fossil fuel burning, all of which are manageable and preventable factors but are underestimated by governmental agencies across the world, despite timely release of monitoring, status, and health impact reports of such diseases by the World Health Organization (WHO) and other international bodies.[4]

The male reproductive structures of plants, pollen grains, as aeroallergen are well studied across the world and are the primary causative agent of pollen allergy or pollinosis, continuously increasing in these changing climatic conditions. Pollinosis encompasses allergic responses such as rhinitis (hay fever) and asthma and globally are an increasing public health concern.[5] Apart from inducing asthma and allergic diseases, a high abundance of pollen has also been associated with nonallergic respiratory diseases, such as chronic obstructive pulmonary disease, stroke, myocardial infarction, and even suicide.[6]

The pollen count, pollen abundance, dispersal, and allergenicity are the parameters that are affected by the local climate.[7] With changing climatic conditions, these variables fluctuate as the phenology is affected. The total allergenicity is not the same throughout the year (major allergens are few and minor allergens constitute more than 50%). The concentrations of airborne pollen or spores and durations of exposure to these allergens have been found to be important factors influencing the exacerbation of allergic symptoms.[8] Pollen grains or plant-derived paucimicronic components (such as stem particles, trichome parts, plant debris) carry allergens that behave as easily respirable particles that can produce allergic symptoms. These plant-derived particles also interact with air pollution (particulate matter, ozone) to modulate the allergenicity, in turn leading to increased airway sensitization.[9]

Pollen grains are produced by flowering plants (angiosperms) and gymnosperms (naked seed plants). Of the 250,000 well-identified and detailed pollen-producing plant species, fewer than 100 are known to induce pollinosis. Among these, pollen grain dispersal mechanisms such as pollination from anemophilous or wind-pollinated plants are the most potent allergen sources, whereas pollens from entomophilous or insect-pollinated plants are known to cause fewer allergic symptoms based on a type I hypersensitivity mechanism.[10] Pollen grains or subparticles less than 2.5 to 10 μm readily enter the human body via upper respiratory tract mucosa for eliciting allergic sensitization. The critical threshold pollen concentration expressed as grains per cubic meter of air required to elicit symptoms of seasonal allergic rhinitis varies for different plant taxa: for grasses, the reported value is 50; for *Olea*, 400; and 1 to ~50 for *Ambrosia* pollen.[11,12] Pollen allergy is also linked with food-allergic disorders, on account of cross reactivity, so any change in pollen abundance and distribution may indirectly affect this condition too.[13-15]

Several studies are oriented toward assessing the adverse effects of increasing temperature and increased CO_2 on phenology regarding productivity, especially for staple and cash crops. Surface pollen records have been widely used for interpretation of fossil pollen history and reconstructions of vegetation and climate in the past.[16] Nonetheless, there are only sparse data on the direct correlations among climate changes, pollen seasons, and allergic sensitizations, because this would require long-term detailed pollen counts and meteorologic monitoring, with simultaneous recording of the clinical data of the resident population of the study site.

The present article highlights the impact of these 3 major risk factors on pollen production, pollen seasons, and altered allergenic content as reported in various studies, with a focus on India and Southeast Asia.

NCDs are man-made disorders related to adoption of unhealthy lifestyles (also unhealthy diet, physical inactivity, and increasing tobacco/alcohol consumption, especially at an early age) in line with the increased urbanization, especially in developing regions such as Southeast Asia.[17,18]

To create urban areas, the green vegetation cover is eroded, land-use changes, human settlement induces microclimatic changes, and this leads to unmatched levels of air quality caused by anthropogenic emissions such as industrial pollution, vehicular traffic, fossil fuels for energy, and cooking fuels for domestic use.[19] The major contributors to air pollution worldwide are the transport emissions in cities, associated with health implications such as respiratory and cardiovascular diseases.[20] The impact of these climate events has already been documented on agricultural crop productivity, natural species diversity and distribution, and other ecosystem services such as flowering time and pollination.

ANTHROPOGENIC ACTIVITY LEADING TO CLIMATE CHANGE: MUCH TO BE UNDERSTOOD

The Mother Land Earth provides the basics for living through the availability of food, freshwater, and multiple other ecosystem services, as well as rich biodiversity. Humans use more than 70% of the global, ice-free land surface.[21] Massive deforestation leads to urbanization and industrialization, population explosion and resulting enhanced transportation and associated increasing vehicular pollution have only eroded the environment but not renewed it at the same rate. Primarily burning of fossil fuels such as coal and oil that have formed over millions of years through photosynthesis-based trapping of carbon is reverting to atmospheric carbon in a shorter time period, adding to the already increased level induced by anthropogenic activity. Second is the massive deforestation leading to unexpected higher levels of carbon in the atmosphere (acting as a sink). Primary emissions from industries and vehicles, secondary emissions and photochemical oxidation, and the concentrations of various air pollutants such as reactive trace gases and aerosols such as ozone, nitrogen, sulfur oxides, and soot have greatly increased, especially in heavily populated and agricultural environments around the globe.[22] The ever-increasing population continuously supported by improved agriculture and forestry productivity in the Anthropocene era has continuously and abruptly led to environmental variation such as change in biodiversity and vegetation, air quality, precipitation duration, and temperature recordings on local, regional, and global scales as climate change events.[22] The Intergovernmental Panel on Climate Change Reports[23,24] document evidence of increased CO_2 concentrations and other greenhouse gases leading to a higher frequency of extreme climate events and being involved in the exchange of energy, water, and aerosols between the land surface and atmosphere and defining climatic conditions. As a consequence of anthropogenic emissions, the planet Earth is facing an increased greenhouse effect leading to global warming, unanticipated climatic events such as extreme heat waves, temperature extremes, shrinking glaciers, forest fires, droughts, and floods, all of which put human health at risk. Paleoclimatic studies have clearly recorded that, within the late Quaternary period, the Holocene (»11,600 years to the present) has witnessed a highly variable climate.[25]

PREVALENCE AND ECONOMIC IMPACT OF NONCOMMUNICABLE DISEASES CAUSED BY CLIMATE CHANGE

According to various timely estimates released by WHO, NCDs had killed 38 million and 41 million people by the years 2012 and 2016, respectively, an undesired but real scenario that is still increasing.[26] NCD deaths have occurred at the highest rate in the WHO Southeast Asia region, from 6.7 million to 8.5 million from 2000 to 2012, and in the western Pacific region, from 8.6 to 10.9 million. During 2011 to 2025, cumulative economic losses caused by NCDs under a business-as-usual scenario in low-income and middle-income countries have been estimated at nearly US$7 trillion as against the estimated annual US$11.2 billion cost of implementing impactful interventions to reduce the NCD burden.[27] Five years from now, (2025) globally NCDs will be account-able for 70% of all deaths, of which 85% will be in developing countries, especially low-income and middle-income countries.[26–28]

PREVALENCE OF RESPIRATORY DISORDERS

A large body of epidemiologic studies have been revealing a general increase in both the incidence and the prevalence of respiratory diseases, including allergic rhinitis (hay fever) and asthma.[1] During the last 60 years, there has been an increase in the epidemic prevalence of allergic disorders, which is expected to reach up to 4 billion in the 2050s.[29] Asthma, allergic rhinitis, atopic dermatitis, and inhalant sensi-tization have been appropriately referred to as the first wave of the epidemic of the twenty-first century, which will become a pandemic comparable with infectious diseases.[30–33]

HOW CLIMATE CHANGE AND AIR POLLUTION AFFECT HUMAN HEALTH

The undesired impacts on human health caused by the combination of climate change and air pollution have become the defining issues for policy makers.[34] Air pollution, climate change, and reduced biodiversity caused by urban lifestyles are presenting threats to human health with unfavorable effects on a variety of chronic disorders such as respiratory and cardiovascular diseases.[35] The constant exposure to pollut-ants and the reduced biodiversity in urban settings have led to limited plant, animal, and microbial interaction, which in turn is causing immune dysfunction and impaired immune tolerance in humans compared with rural populations exposed to the same levels of pollution but residing in habitats rich in flora and fauna. Air pollution is strongly associated with climate change.[36]

A recent position statement on climate change and health impacts from the Euro-pean Respiratory Society (ERS) was developed after a workshop co-organized by the Health and Environment Network (HENVINET) Project and the American Thoracic Society. The position statement highlights climate-related health impacts, including deaths and acute morbidity caused by heat waves, increased frequency of acute cardiorespiratory events caused by higher concentrations of ground-level ozone, changes in the frequency of respiratory diseases caused by transboundary particle pollution, and altered spatial and temporal distribution of allergens (pollens, molds, and mites) and some infectious disease vectors.[37–39] According to the WHO, every year 3 million people die prematurely because of outdoor air pollution, which is heav-iest in major cities of Asia, Africa, and Latin America.[35]

Fossil fuel and transportation are the main sources of air pollution (eg, sulfur oxide and nitrous oxides) released into the atmosphere, leading to health problems, poor air quality, and acid rain. Air pollutants show these effects by causing direct cellular injury or by inducing intracellular signaling pathways and transcription factors that are known to be sensitive to oxidative stress. Outdoor air pollution exacerbates asthma in people who already have the condition.[2]

PREVALENCE OF ASTHMA

A global study found that from 9 million to 23 million and from 5 million to 10 million annual asthma emergency room visits globally in 2015 could be attributable to O_3 and particulate matter (PM) with a diameter of 2.5 μm or less (PM2.5), respectively, representing 8% to 20% and 4% to 9% of the annual number of global visits, respectively The top 3 countries for both asthma incidence and prevalence in Asia are India, China, and Indonesia, driven largely by population size; nearly half (48%) of estimated O_3-attributable and more than half (56%) of PM2.5-attributable asthma emergency room visits were estimated in Southeast Asia (including India), and western Pacific regions.[40] Of all countries globally, India and China had the most estimated asthma emergency room visits attributable to total air pollution concentrations, respectively contributing 23% and 10% of global asthma emergency room visits estimated to be associated with O_3, 30% and 12% for PM2.5%, and 15% and 17% for nitrogen dioxide (NO_2). The national pediatric asthma incidence that may be attributable to anthropogenic PM2.5 was estimated to be 57% in India, 51% in China, and more than 70% in Bangladesh. PM2.5 has been causatively linked to the most premature deaths. Acute respiratory tract infections, asthma, chronic obstructive pulmonary disease, exacerbations of preexisting obstructive airway disease, and lung cancer are proven adverse respiratory effects of air pollution.[2]

The drastic changes in climate and air quality have a quantifiable impact on the morbidity of respiratory diseases.[38] An easily understandable tabular association of environmental changes with impacts on health systems is presented in **Table 1**.[36] Climate change as been found to affect human health via 3 pathways. Primarily, the direct unpredictable impacts are caused by the associated extreme weather events

Table 1
Climate change and impact on the biosphere

Climate Events	Agriculture, Forestry	Human Health Impact
Heavy precipitation events: frequency increases over most areas	Damage to crops; soil erosion, inability to cultivate land, waterlogging of soils; adverse effects on quality of surface and groundwater; contamination of water supply	Deaths, injuries, infectious diseases, allergies, and dermatitis from floods and landslides
Area affected by drought	Land degradation, lower yields/crop damage and failure; livestock deaths; land degradation; more widespread water stress	Increased risk of food and water shortage; increased risk of water-borne and food-borne diseases; cardiovascular disorders
Number of intense tropical cyclones	Damage to crops; windthrow of trees; power outages cause disruption of public water supply	Increased risk of water-borne and food-borne diseases; asthma
Incidence of extreme highsea level	Salinization of irrigation and well water; decreased freshwater availability caused by saltwater intrusion	Increase in stress-related disease; other allergic conditions

Adapted from D'Amato G, Vitale C, Rosario N et al. Climate change, allergy and asthma, and the role of tropical forests. World Allergy Organ J 2017;10(1):11; with permission.

of heat and drought, heavy rainfall, flooding, and cyclones. The consequences of the primary events are witnessed through their impacts on natural ecosystems, agricultural productivity, species migration, and through changing the burden and pattern of distribution of vector-borne, water-borne, and food-borne diseases. In addition, climate change may affect health indirectly, via social institutions, resulting in health-related unemployment, undernutrition, mental ill-health, violence, and conflict.[3]

CLIMATE CHANGE AFFECTING BIOSPHERE

A large number of evidence-based studies[22,36,41,42] have explored and detailed the indirect unending impacts of climatic events on various components of the biosphere, such as:

- Altered agricultural productivity
- Changing patterns of natural species diversity and distribution
- Migration of pests and vectors affecting pollination
- Easy entry of new invasive plant species to new areas
- Phenology (ie, ecosystem factors such as flowering time and onset, duration, and intensity of pollination, fruiting pattern)
- Altered allergenicity of pollen and fungal spores

The primary indirect effect is from the spatial increase in temperature caused by greenhouse gas concentrations varying with geography. Water vapor is the primary greenhouse gas at the equator, creating a warm, humid climate, so the influence of CO_2 is less pronounced, whereas, at the poles and in deserts, the effect is impactful. Likewise, the winters at northern latitudes are colder and drier and will get warm faster because of CO_2. The variation arising from anthropogenic greenhouse gases is driving extreme climatic events, with a strong influence on plant biology worldwide.[43] The second direct factor affecting all aspects of plants' life cycles is the increasing atmospheric CO_2 concentration, which affects plant growth. Atmospheric CO_2 is the raw material for terrestrial green plant photosynthesis, and thus it represents the first molecular link in the food chain of the entire Earth. The impact of this factor is species and tissue development dependent. Under optimal conditions of temperature and light intensity, the rate of photosynthesis markedly increases.[44]

PHENOLOGY AND CLIMATE CHANGE

The mechanism of flowering is primarily dependent on photoperiodism: the effect of day length (periodicity), temperature, CO_2, and water content. A critical duration of light in long-day plants and dark in short-day plants is required by different species. The plant pigment phytochrome in its 2 forms phytochrome red (Pr_{660}) and phytochrome far red (Pfr_{730}) perceives the light stimulus, leading to hormonal changes and induction of flowering. Addressing the effect of these environmental factors on flowering events such as time of day of anthesis and flowering time (duration from germination till flowering) is essential to understand the adaptation of plants/crops to changing climatic conditions. Flowering is the decisive phase determining reproductive success and seed set in the later life cycle of plants emerging after the vegetative growth phase.[45]

Phenology is the study of effects of climatic factors on the life cycle events of animals and plants. The various reproductive events in the life cycles of flowering plants are termed phenoevents, such as the onset of flowering and fruiting and seed dispersal, and they follow a seasonal pattern. Phenoevents serve as sensor-indicators for climate change, of migration of species to higher elevations and altitudes.[14,46] A noteworthy example is the accurate long-term records on the phenology of flowering time of cherry blossom (*Prunus jamasakura*) in Japan for the past 1200 years, coinciding with the cherry blossom festival from time immemorial. The flowers blossom an average of 7 days earlier compared with records before 1970.[47] For a nearly 50-year dataset from a Europe-wide network (1951–1996), the International Phenological Gardens reported an increase in annual growing season by approximately 11 days.[48]

A detailed compilation of the effects of 2 environmental factors, increased CO_2 and temperature, alone or in combination, on the flowering times of a wide range of flowering species and specific ecosystems has been analyzed and reported.[45] As per the records of flowering time, pollen data, and herbaria, for perennials, flowering time had advanced, with an annual advancement of 9 days and a delay of up to 16 days being recorded.[49,50] On average, flowering time advanced by 4 to 6 days per 1°C according to historical data for more than 400 plant species and deciduous trees at decadal time scale for the past few centuries. For annual grasses, flowering time has been delayed up to 6 days under increased CO_2 levels, whereas, in combination with warming effects, advancement of 2 to 4 days has been reported. For C4 weeds, an advanced flowering of 10 to 15 days has been reported under high CO_2 concentrations, whereas, for desert shrubs under high-temperature regimes, flowering has been advanced by 20 to 41 days.

IMPACT ON PHENOLOGY IN INDIA

An overall delay in flowering has been recorded for legumes. In India, the data for different varieties of peach, apple, and kiwi growing in hilly regions show a considerable delay in flowering in 2008 owing to low winter temperatures, whereas in 2006 and 2009 it was early because of warmer winters.[51] In the Uttaranchal state, located in the upper hilly region (Himalayas) of north India, the most notable evidence is the flowering of *Rhododendron* spp, which have been flowering 15 days earlier with small flowers in relation to 15 to 20 years ago because of changing rainfall patterns.[42]

C3/C4 ANATOMY: ADAPTATION TO HIGH TEMPERATURE AND INCREASED CO_2

The shift in C3 and C4 plant types seems to be related to change in moisture and atmospheric CO_2, with lower moisture and CO_2 levels favoring the C4 plant types. The oscillating climate has resulted in mean temperatures in the tropics increasing by at least 1°C to 2°C as a result of increase in atmospheric CO_2, methane, and other greenhouse gases.[52] General circulation models predict an intensification of the Indian summer monsoon as a consequence of the increased temperature,[42] which is consistent with the paleoclimate record. These climatic changes can be expected to favor the expansion of C3 vegetation more than C4 vegetation for several reasons. Higher CO_2 levels would enhance photosynthesis rates in C3 plants to a greater extent than in C4 plants. Higher temperatures would reduce the incidence of frost and promote the survival of C3 forest plants. Higher precipitation and soil moisture would favor the growth of C3 plants. Thus, the montane evergreen forest can be expected to expand into the grasslands, whereas C3 grasses and herbs could potentially replace C4 grasses in the grasslands.[42] However, a counterargument is that C4 plants will have better adaptability for long-term survival in drier conditions because of being able to cope better with water stress and higher temperatures. An increase in C4 plants may result in ecosystems with more allergenic plant species.[53]

IMPACT OF CLIMATE ON POLLEN ALLERGY

Aerobiology deals with the study of the impact of the bioparticulate matter present in the Earth's atmosphere on human health. The bioparticulates described to cause allergic symptoms are pollen grains, fungal spores, insect debris, house dust mites, animal dander, chemicals, foods, and so forth.[54] Among all these agents, pollen grains and fungal spores are the predominant allergens in the air worldwide. Climate change is related to aeroallergens, in particular pollen, because various climate change events affect the phenological response of plant life cycles, leading to increased and faster growth, earlier start of pollen seasons, greater pollen production, and enhanced allergenic response in susceptible individuals.

The word pollen is derived from a Latin word meaning fine flour or dust.[55] The pollen is the minute vital part of flowering plants and has special morphology and function. Pollens are single cells representing the microgametophytes of seed plants destined to produce male gametes (sperm cells).[56] Pollen allergens are classified into size classes and generally belong to the coarse fraction of air particulate matter (particle diameters >10 μm), but fungal spores and pollen fragments are also found in fine particulate matter (<2.5 μm; PM2.5), which can penetrate deep into the human respiratory tract and alveolar regions of the lung.[22] Pollen allergens are classified into size classes as detailed in **Table 2**.[57] Most of the living angiosperms have pollen grains in the range of 25 to 100 μm. Pollen of the families Boraginaceae, Piperaceae, Crypteroniaceae, and Cunoniaceae have low size ranges. Monocots have been reported to produce grains in the size range of 15 to 80 μm. Pollen of anemophilous plants are small, whereas those of entomophilous plants are large.[58–73]

CLIMATE AND POLLEN MORPHOLOGY

The wall of pollen is primarily divided into an inner intine and an outer sculptured exine. The inner layer is rich in cellulose and the outer wall is composed of sporopollenin, a tough, resistant biopolymer enabling the pollen to withstand extremely high temperatures of up to 3000°C, strong acids, and harmful radiation.[56,58] Chemically, intine is composed of cellulose and lignin. Chemically, the sporopollenin resembles lignin and is a polymerization product of hydrocarbons, carotenoid, and carotenoid esters. The pollen wall imparts protection to sperm while the pollen grain is traveling in the air from the anther to the stigma; it protects the vital genetic material from drying out. When pollen lands on a pistil of the same flower or another flower, the pollen germinates and a pollen tube emerges, which grows downward in the pistil to reach the

Table 2 Size-based categorization of pollen grains	
Size (μm)	**Category**
<10	Very small pollens (*Myosotis*)
10–25	Small pollens (*Salix*)
25–50	Medium pollens (*Quercus*)
50–100	Large pollens (*Zea*)
100–200	Very large pollens (*Cucurbita*)
>200	Giant pollens (*Mirabilis*)

From Morphologic Encyclopedia of Palynology by Gerhard Kremp © 1965 The Arizona Board of Regents. Reprinted by permission of the University of Arizona Press.

ovule (female gametophyte), fertilize it, and begin a new generation. The entire process involves a variety of stored compounds, with glycoproteins predominating in the mature pollen grain.[74] Pollen apertures are named for the various wall modifications, which may involve thinning, ridges, and pores. They serve as an exit for the pollen's contents and allow shrinking and swelling of the grain caused by changes in osmotic potential of the surrounding medium. Morphologically, it is an aperture or a thinning of exine (except in operculate apertures) where the intine is thickened, except in the poplar plant (*Populus*), which lacks them.

Pollen grains primarily cause asthma, allergic rhinitis, and allergic conjunctivitis in atopic patients.[75] The distribution and prevalence of pollen allergy are subject to both geographic and chronologic variations.[76] Pollen allergy is a topic for studying the interrelationship between air pollution and allergic respiratory diseases such as rhinitis and asthma.[9,77]

Pollen grains are more sensitive at the early stages of development (anther wall development, microsporogenesis, and microgametogenesis) than at later stages (pollen maturation and anther dehiscence) or during the progamic phase (pollen hydration, germination, growth and guidance of the pollen tube). During maturation, pollen grains undergo various degrees of cellular dehydration before and/or after an anther dehiscence. The water content of pollen grains decreases to 40% to 58% and pollen becomes physiologically dormant until landing on a receptive stigma.[78] The ready-to-disperse pollen thus has a reduced metabolic activity to ensure long-term viability in the external environment. Bicellular pollen is generally more dehydrated and less metabolically active than tricellular pollen. Temperature variations have a strong effect on pollen desiccation. Stacks of rough endoplasmic reticulum are largely dissociated in heat-stressed pollen, consequently affecting protein processing and secretion.[79] Heat stress induces adverse effects on dehiscence of anthers and discharge of pollen in rice.[80–90]

POLLINOSIS AND POLLEN ALLERGENS

Allergen release from pollen is a prerequisite for sensitization and elicitation of the allergic symptoms in humans. A 2-route process has been suggested: first, outside the individual organism when pollen grains are spreading through the atmosphere, and, second, on reaching and in contact with the mucosal surface of the upper respiratory tract. Aeroallergenic particles such as pollen and plant/pollen-derived submicronic (<10 µm) and paucimicronic (<1 µm) particles can reach the lower airways, eliciting allergic symptoms in susceptible people. These particles are mainly composed of starch granules and polysaccharide particles, which may be absent in mature pollen.[91]

The most important outdoor sources of allergens are pollen grains from anemophilous plants, including trees, grasses, and weeds. To increase the chance of fertilization, wind-pollinated plants have evolved characteristic features such as small, dehydrated pollen with good aerodynamic properties that allow dissemination over hundreds of kilometers.

The presence of allergens in pollen and their levels of expression may vary depending on plant species, changing climate, maturation stage, and environmental factors (pollution). Because of changes in climatic conditions, observations on diurnal and seasonal prevalence become very important because information gained in this way has direct applications to treating patients with hay fever.[92]

Climate change affects aeroallergens and, in particular, plant allergens, as reported by several experimental and epidemiologic studies. As described earlier in the article, climate change interacts with the increased concentration of atmospheric CO_2 to boost plant growth, which in turn leads to increased pollen production, affecting anther dehiscence and pollen dispersal and transport, accelerating the start and duration of the pollen season, along with the emergence of new pollen species in new locations that are not endemic to the specific area.[2] The onset, duration, and intensity of pollination, the fruiting patterns and sporulation of fungi, along with the allergen content and allergenicity of pollen grains, fungal spores, and other bioparticulates become altered under changing climatic conditions.[22,36,93] Global warming–led increased CO_2 in the atmosphere is reported to alter the start, duration, and intensity of the pollen season along with the rate of asthma exacerbations arising from respiratory infections and cold air inhalation.[93]

ALLERGENIC PLANTS, CLIMATE CHANGE, AND POLLUTANTS AFFECTING ALLERGENICITY

In order to monitor the occurrence and abundances of pollen grains in the ambient air for early warning of allergic diseases as well as other health risks, a limited number of studies have been conducted in Southeast Asia.[6] A planned routine study is investigating the diurnal, seasonal, and annual fluctuations in the concentrations of atmospheric pollen, especially from allergenic plants, in relation to the meterological factors that will always be the governing factor in the correct diagnosis and therapeutic treatment of patients with pollen-induced respiratory allergic disorders.[80] With a continuously changing climate, such information is essential for timely prevention and better patient outcomes in this era of customized precision treatment. Classic relevant studies of this topic are reviewed and highlighted later.

Reports from the Australian Institute of Health and Welfare (AIHW) show that, in 2014 to 2015, nearly 1 in 5 Australians had pollen allergy, which amounts to 4.5 million citizens, mainly comprising the working population.[94] Grasses are the major aeroallergens in Australia, with varying clinical implications. The indigenous vegetation includes plant species of *Eucalyptus*, *Acacia*, and *Sorthum* grass along with introduced self-thriving northern hemisphere species such as ragweed, birch, and exotic invasive species expanding their range under the changing climate conditions.[95]

For the available sporadic studies, pollen monitoring has been restricted to sites within the coastal state capital cities, where most of the Australian population resides.[96,97]

No national level prospective planned studies encompassing aerobiological monitoring, impact of climate change, along with increased hospital visits have been performed. Grasses have been showing increased atmospheric pollen concentrations resulting in the strong, consistent appearance of allergic asthma symptoms leading to heightened primary care or emergency department visits during peak pollen seasons. Because the seasonality is affected in an unpredictable manner by anthropogenic climate change, urbanization and global warming future strategies for prevention and treatment are difficult to plan. Ironically, little research has been focused on studying the impact of climate change on timing and duration of the grass pollen season in Australasia.[98] The available pollen indices published on the Internet are not based on current local pollen data and have been found to be misleading, risking public health.[98] It is disappointing that research on pollen aerobiology in a developed country such as Australia is lagging.

The necessity and importance of aerobiological surveys was clear after a Melbourne thunderstorm asthma event in November 2016 that resulted in 10 deaths and 9000 patients requiring hospital emergency department visits for asthma attacks.[99] Because of the lack of planned studies, a national pollen monitoring service within a partnership known as the AusPollen project has been advocated to fill the knowledge gap and attempt to map allergenic pollen and fungi distributions and correlate thee with respiratory allergy incidents and likely hospital visits.[14] However, few modern pollen monitoring programs use automated counting instruments capable of integrating with transdisciplinary research areas such as geospatial science climate change science, molecular allergology, and mathematical modeling of pollen transport and dispersal.[43,98]

A study assessed atmospheric pollen concentrations and the clinical grass pollen season and grass pollen peaks over a long time period (1995–2013) for various cities in Australia, such as Brisbane, Canberra, Darwin, Hobart, Melbourne, and Sydney. Climate, weather, and meteorological variables have been identified as influencing factors for the pollen season and larger-scale climate fluctuations events such as the El Niño. The delayed and lessened 1997 to 1998 grass pollen season in Brisbane corresponded with a 12-month to 14-month El Niño effect that started early in 1997, which was associated with below-average rainfall in eastern subtropical Queensland, and this is an added dimension of climate change impact.[96]

THUNDERSTORM-ASSOCIATED ASTHMA EPIDEMICS IN POLLEN SEASONS

The Intergovernmental Panel on Climate Change Reports[23,24] document evidence of increased concentrations of CO_2 and other greenhouse gases leading to a higher frequency of extreme climate events. Thunderstorms present a unique sum of environmental factors that lead to increase aeroallergen burden.[100] Some of the first observation-based evidence regarding thunderstorms and asthma outbreaks was reported from East Birmingham Hospital (Birmingham, United Kingdom) on July 6 and 7, 1983, leading to increased hospital visits.[101] In the United Kingdom, a large number of thunderstorms (those with a large number of lightning discharges, such as electromagnetic impulses or sferics), probably after days of high grass pollen counts, have been associated with heightened emergency department visits, especially among child and adult asthmatics.[100]

The 2016 asthma epidemic in Melbourne, Victoria, represented an unusual association of environmental factors, such as prevailing weather wind conditions and torrential rain combined with a high pollen count (the dominant aeroallergen was grass pollen with density $>100/m^3$), resulting a city-wide spread of huge pollen and pollen-derived particles of respirable size. Melbourne was unprepared for the rapid response needed to combat the growing medical emergencies, and this day tested the capacity of Melbourne's health system.[99]

The focus of the European and Mediterranean Plant Protection Organization is the alien, invasive, and noxious plant species *Ambrosia artemisiifolia* L. (common ragweed), which has highly allergenic pollen.[1] Ragweed, a native of North America, has been invading large areas of South America and Europe for the last few decades and has been identified as a major contributor to severe respiratory allergic diseases. The plant has been rightly described as successful dominant species in abandoned lands even under severe ecophysiologic conditions of extreme and unpredictable environments.[102]

The species has naturalized across Europe at a rapid rate, and accounts for high sensitization rates. The most important allergen is named Amb a 1. In another German health study, immunoglobulin E sensitization rates to *A artemisiifolia* were 8.2% among German adults, with the prevalence increasing even at very low concentrations (5–10 pollen grains per cubic meter of air), which were sufficient to trigger allergic reactions in sensitive patients. Sikoparija and colleagues[103] reported increased prevalence and incidence of asthma with this new allergen at a high frequency compared with other pollen types. The effect of doubling CO_2 levels led to a 61% increase in the amount of pollen, whereas another study reported an increase in major allergen concentration, Amb a 1, with increasing CO_2 with no change in total protein level.[14,104] Furthermore, ragweed pollen collected along high-traffic roads showed a higher allergenicity than pollen sampled in vegetated areas, probably caused by traffic-related pollution. The overall impact will be altered pollen season timing and load, and hence change in exposure.[36]

About a third of the airborne pollen increase is caused by on-going seed dispersal, irrespective of climate change. The remaining two-thirds are related to climate and land-use changes that will extend ragweed habitat suitability in northern and eastern Europe and increase pollen production in established ragweed areas owing to increasing CO_2.[1,14]

There is a long-term record of 27 years (1981–2007) of pollen counts, meteorological factors, and clinical data for western Liguaria (northwest Italy), thanks to a detailed cause-effect study highlighting the effect of climate variables on the allergic sensitization rate. The duration of pollen seasons was recorded to lengthen for *Parietaria* (85 days), olive (18 days), and cypress (18 days), with an advancement in their start dates (**Table 3**). Except for the grasses, the pollen load increased for the other 2 stated species. The noteworthy analysis was the constant increase in pollen sensitization through the year with the increasing pollen load, whereas sensitization to house dust mite remained stable.[7]

SOUTH ASIA

Only scant information is available from Southeast Asian countries, including India. The airspora in Southeast Asia, a tropical region, mainly comprises trees and shrubs flourishing year-round, with an abundance of ferns. There is no distinct definable major flowering season for plants compared with temperate countries.[105–114]

In an investigational study based on the medical data records of patients visiting University Hospital in Gyeonggi Province Seoul, Korea, from 1999 to 2008, a possible correlation of skin test positivity results and hospitalization of patients with tree pollen allergy affected temporally by meteorologic variations is reported. Controlling for the air pollutant levels during the study period of months April to July, a contributory

Table 3															
Start and end dates and durations of the pollen seasons of 5 allergenic plants under consideration (5-year averages)															
	1981–1985			1986–1990			1991–1995			1996–2000			2001–2007		
Pollen	S	E	D	S	E	D	S	E	D	S	E	D	S	E	D
Birch	71	165	91	42	148	76	57	141	81	45	133	104	44	145	79
Cypress	309	146	178	305	96	154	326	61	112	303	121	161	300	138	196
Parietaria	107	291	219	55	279	217	144	317	270	33	296	275	24	342	304
Olive	151	202	56	124	267	78	118	226	109	120	182	65	105	180	74
Grass	144	230	97	102	257	105	115	229	106	136	216	99	118	214	87

Abbreviations: D, duration; E, end; S, start.

Adapted from Ariano R, Canonica GW, Passalacqua G. Possible role of climate changes in variations in pollen seasons and allergic sensitizations during 27 years. Ann Allergy Asthma Immunol 2010;104(3):215–22; with permission.

association of increasing minimum temperature in March (preflowering period) with higher pollen counts leading to increase tree pollen sensitization and hence more hospital visits has been suggested. In Korea, pollen levels of trees are higher than those of grass/weeds, with yearly tree pollen accounting for 95% in the spring season, which extends from March to May, as did the study period.[115]

Among several cities in Korea for which pollen counts are monitored, Japanese cedar (JC) pollen was detected only in Jeju as the most frequent sensitizer among outdoor aeroallergens. The sensitization rates for JC pollen are much higher (33.8%) in Jeju than in Seoul (1.1%) and Suwon (0.7%). A first-of-its-kind study on pollinosis to JC pollen in Jeju City, South Korea, a temperate geographic zone, has been reported. The JC has been the dominant tree species as a windbreak for the tangerine orchard industry. A study on school children from Jeju in northern region (NR) and Seogwipo in southern region (SR) locations on aeroallergen sensitization showed the highest sensitization to *Dermatophagoides pteronyssinus* (35.8%), followed by *Dermatophagoides farinae* (26.2%), and JC pollen (17.6%). The JC pollen season was estimated from 2011 to 2013.

In the SR, the JC pollen season lasted for 47 days in 2011, 72 days in 2012, and 95 days in 2013, whereas in the NR it lasted for 43 days in 2011, 65 days in 2012, and 65 days in 2013. The JC pollen season started earlier and lasted longer in the SR than in the NR (see **Table 3**). For pollen counts measured on the peak days, the level of JC pollen in the atmosphere in the SR was estimated to be 2 to 8 times higher than that in the NR. Overall, the JC pollen season in Jeju can be considered to be from late January to mid-April. A case of JC pollinosis was defined as one with pollinosis symptoms present during the JC efflorescence season in a patient sensitized to JC pollen. The rate of sensitization to JC among schoolchildren in Jeju has undoubtedly increased over time, and, as postulated earlier, a higher rate of sensitization in the older participants might be related to their longer cumulative environmental exposure to pollen. Interestingly, an age-related increment in sensitization was observed in the Seogwipo residents but not in the Jeju residents. This finding could be related to the difference in climate between the 2 geographic regions. The sensitization rate for JC pollen has been increasing year by year. In 1998, the sensitization rate for JC pollen was 9.7%, which increased to 18.2% in 2008, 17.6% in 2010, and 24.4% in 2013 among schoolchildren in Jeju (unpublished data from the Environmental Health Center). Why is the rate of sensitization to JC pollen increasing? During the JC pollen season, there was a difference in the mean temperature between the geographic regions. The mean temperature during the main efflorescence season for JC pollen was higher by 2.0°C in February and by 1.9°C in March in Seogwipo than in Jeju. It is hypothesized that there may be 2 ways that global climate change could influence human health: an indirect effect by increasing the average temperature, and a direct effect caused by CO_2-induced stimulation of photosynthesis and plant growth.[14,15] Warmer weather evokes earlier flowering, more effective pollen scattering in the air, and a prolonged efflorescence season.[16–18] Monitoring has shown an increasing mean temperature in Jeju since 1990.[19] The current study supports the hypothesis that any global warming, especially in the flowering season, might increase the rate of sensitization to JC pollen in future, which results in a greater prevalence of pollinosis. The prevalence of symptomatic JC pollinosis is estimated to be half that of JC pollen sensitization, regardless of the region. This study is the first to address the relationship between pollen counts, sensitization rate, and the prevalence of JC pollinosis in Jeju, Korea.[116]

A 6-year study (2008–2013) from Seoul, Korea, evaluated the changes in pollen count and retrospectively examined the Skin Prick Test (SPT) results of 4442 patients of an asthma clinic. Meteorologic observations suggest no significant annual increase in pollen count for trees, grasses, and weeds. Clinically, the skin positivity rates in relation to pollen from grasses, weeds, and trees increased significantly during the study. The SPT rates increased significantly in response to pollen from walnut, popular, elm, and alder. Further, there was a significant correlation between the annual rate of change in pollen count and the rate of change in skin positivity rate for oak and Japanese hop. Therefore, there must be a climate-related increased increase in pollen count for the last 2 of these plants, whereas, for the 4 trees, despite no increase in pollen count, SPT increased positively, indicating there might be some enhancement in pollen allergenicity or more efficient pollen dispersal and duration of suspension in the air.[9,76]

In Japan after World War II, from early 1950 to early 1960, an undesired consequence arising from the mass afforestation program was the planting of 4.6 billion straight and tall JC trees (Cryptomeria japonica; ie, sugi), covering nearly 18% of the total land area of Japan. These trees were considered an ideal construction material but, after heavy tariff reduction in 1964, imported wood put the native foresters out of business. As a result, most of the sugi trees are standing abandoned, growing taller each year and producing more pollen year after year. The yellow green dust or JC pollen is scattered across the whole of Japan with the exception of Hokkaido and the Okinawan islands. Cedar pollen released from male flowers of sugi trees is dispersed in large quantities, over long distances (up to 100 km in some cases), remains airborne for more than 12 hours (prolonged season), and has been positively linked to uninterrupted increasing prevalence and severity of sugi pollinosis. The total JC pollen count is continuously increasing because there was a significant difference from 1995 to 2013 compared with the initial period of monitoring, 1965 to 1994 ($P<.05$). Sugi pollinosis was first reported in 1963. Seasonal Allergic Rhinitis (SAR) caused by JC pollen has been rightly declared to be the national affliction of Japan. The prevalence rate of SAR in Tokyo schoolchildren has been found to be extremely high by the International Study of Asthma and Allergies in Childhood (ISAAC). The pollen season is January to February. The temperature in these months influences the start of sugi pollen production and the pollen season. To worsen the conditions further, pollen release from the Japanese cypress (Chamaecyparis obtusa) follows, causing SAR, in the months of April and May, immediately after the release of JC pollen. JC and cypress pollens are considered to contain several components that cross react with each other, leading to additional severity in 70% of patients with sugi pollinosis. Therefore allergic symptoms can last for as long as 4 months, from February to May. Hot summers usually affect sugi trees, promoting flower bud development and increasing pollen production; meanwhile, cool summers have the opposite effects. Ironically, warm summers (higher mean temperature) have been affected by the side effects of global warming and climate change affecting plant morphology, flowering phenology, and pollen production. Climate change in Japan has been more severe, with temperatures increasing by an average of 1.158 C during the past 100 years. As such, the length of the sugi pollinosis season has increased since 1995, leading to increased prevalence, as stated earlier, and this is in line with the various reported epidemiologic studies highlighting global climate change–led temperature increase correlating with the increasing number of pollen-induced respiratory allergies. Pollution in the form of Asian dust (AD) and urban particulate matter (PM2.5) are risk factors for sugi pollinosis. AD is a seasonal phenomenon affecting much of eastern Asia, including Japan, and occasionally spreads around the globe, affecting the United States as well.[15] The number of spring dust storms has increased in the last 13 years. The frequency of the storms combined with increased air pollutant concentrations have been reported for adverse health effects such as increased allergic symptoms in Japan and Taipei.

Animal studies have shown that the combination of AD plus JC pollen results in inducing type I hypersensitivity and sensitization in nonatopic or unsensitized atopic people.[117]

CLINICS CARE POINTS

- The incidence of allergic diseases is partially increasing due to climate change with increasing pollen productivity and duration of exposure.

REFERENCES

1. Damialis A, Traidl-Hoffmann C, Treudler R. Climate change and pollen allergies. In: Marselle M, Stadler J, Korn H, et al, editors. Biodiversity and health in the face of climate change. Cham (Switzerland): Springer; 2019.
2. Pawankar R, Wang JY, Wang IJ, et al. Asia pacific association of allergy asthma and clinical immunology white paper 2020 on climate change, air pollution, and biodiversity in asia-pacific and impact on allergic diseases. Asia Pac Allergy 2020;10:e11.
3. Wheeler N, Watts N. Climate change: from science to practice. Curr Environ Health Rep 2018;5:170–8.
4. Schiavoni G, D'Amato G, Afferni C. The dangerous liaison between pollens and pollution in respiratory allergy. Ann Allergy Asthma Immunol 2017;118:269–75.
5. Rasmussen K, Thyrring J, Muscarella R, et al. Climate-change-induced range shifts of three allergenic ragweeds (Ambrosia L.) in Europe and their potential impact on human health. Peer J 2017;5:e3104.
6. Hu W, Wang Z, Huang S, et al. Biological aerosol particles in polluted regions. Curr Pollut Rep 2020;6:65–89.
7. Ariano R, Canonica GW, Passalacqua G. Possible role of climate changes in variations in pollen seasons and allergic sensitizations during 27 years. Ann Allergy Asthma Immunol 2010;104:215–22.
8. Songnuan W, Bunnag C, Soontrapa K, et al. Airborne pollen survey in Bangkok, Thailand: A 35-year update. Asian Pac J Allergy Immunol 2015;33:253–62.
9. D'Amato G, Liccardi G, D'Amato M, et al. The role of outdoor air pollution and climatic changes on the rising trends in respiratory allergy. Respir Med 2001; 95:606–11.
10. Mothes N, Horak F, Valenta R. Transition from a botanical to a molecular classification in tree pollen allergy: implications for diagnosis and therapy. Int Arch Allergy Immunol 2004;135:357–73.
11. Breton MC, Garneau M, Fortier I, et al. Relationship between climate, pollen concentrations of Ambrosia and medical consultations for allergic rhinitis in Montreal, 1994–2002. Sci Total Environ 2006;370:39–50.
12. Florido JF, Delgado PG, de San Pedro B, et al. High levels of Olea Europaea pollen and relation with clinical findings. Int Arch Allergy Immunol 1999;119:133–7.
13. García-Mozo H. Poaceae pollen as the leading aeroallergen worldwide: a review. Allergy 2017;72:1849–58.
14. Katelaris CH, Beggs PJ. Climate change: allergens and allergic diseases. Intern Med J 2018;48:129–34.
15. Park JW. Revised pollen calendar in Korea. Allergy Asthma Immunol Res 2020; 12:171–2.
16. Singh S, Scharf BW, Khandelwal A, et al. Modern pollen-vegetation relationship as an adjunct in the interpretation of fossil pollen records in the Chilka Lagoon, Odisha, India. The Palaeobotanist 2011;60:265–71.

17. Angkurawaranon C, Jiraporncharoen W, Chenthanakij B, et al. Urbanization and non-communicable disease in Southeast Asia: a review of current evidence. Public Health 2014;128:886–95.
18. Eckert S, Kohler S. Urbanization and health in developing countries: a systematic review. World Health Popul 2014;15:7–20.
19. Kumar P, Druckman A, Gallagher J, et al. The nexus between air pollution, green infrastructure and human health. Environ Int 2019;133:105181.
20. Heal MR, Kumar P, Harrison RM. Particles, air quality, policy and health. Chem Soc Rev 2012;41:6606–30.
21. Intergovernmental Panel on Climate Change, IPCC 2019. Summary for policymakers. In: Shukla PR, Skea J, Buendia EC et al editors. Climate change and land: an IPCC special report on climate change, desertification, land degradation, sustainable land management, food security, and greenhouse gas fluxes in terrestrial ecosystems,(in press).
22. Reinmuth-Selzle K, Kampf CJ, Lucas K, et al. Air pollution and climate change effects on allergies in the anthropocene: abundance, interaction, and modification of allergens and adjuvants. Environ Sci Technol 2017;51:4119-41.
23. Hegerl GC, Zwiers FW, Braconnot P, et al. Understanding and attributing climate change. In: Solomon S, Qin D, Manning M, et al, editors. Climate change 2007: the physical science basis, Contribution of the working group I to the fourth assessment report of the intergovernmental panel on climate change. Cambridge (United Kingdom): Cambridge University Press; 2007. p. 663–746.
24. Intergovernmental Panel on Climate Change, IPCC. In: Stocker TF, Qin D, Plattner G-K, et al, editors. Climate Change 2013: the physical science basis. contribution of working group i to the fifth assessment report of the intergovernmental panel on climate change. Cambridge(United Kingdom): Cambridge University Press, United Kingdom and New York, NY, USA; 2013. p. 1535.
25. Kar R, Quamar M. Pollen-based Quaternary palaeoclimatic studies in India: an overview of recent advance. Palynology 2019;43:76–93.
26. Noncommunicable diseases country profiles 2018. Geneva: World Health Organization; 2018. Licence: CC BY-NC-SA 3.0 IGO.
27. Global status report on noncommunicable diseases 2014. Geneva: World Health Organization; 2014.Licence: CC BY-NC-SA 3.0 IGO.
28. Noncommunicable diseases progress monitor 2015. Geneva: World Health Organization; 2014. Licence: CC BY-NC-SA 3.0 IGO.
29. Lötvall J, Pawankar R, Wallace DV, et al. American academy of allergy, asthma & immunology (AAAAI), the American college of allergy, asthma & immunology (ACAAI), the European academy of allergy and clinical immunology (EAACI), and the word allergy organisation (WAO). We call for iCAALL: international collaboration in asthma, allergy and immunology. World Allergy Organ J 2012; 5:139–40.
30. Holgate ST. The epidemic of allergy and asthma. Nature 1999;402:B2–4.
31. Vlahov D, Galea S. Urbanization, urbanicity, and health. J Urban Health 2002;79: S1–12.
32. Prescott S, Allen KJ. Food allergy: riding the second wave of the allergy epidemic. Pediatr Allergy Immunol 2011;22:155–60.
33. Asam C, Hofer H, Wolf M, et al. Tree pollen allergens—an update from a molecular perspective. Allergy 2015;70:1201–11.
34. Paramesh H. Air pollution and allergic airway diseases: social determinants and sustainability in the control and prevention. Indian J Pediatr 2018;85:284–94.

35. Pawankar R. Climate change, air pollution, and biodiversity in Asia Pacific: impact on allergic diseases. Asia Pac Allergy 2019;9:2.
36. D'Amato G, Vitale C, Rosario N, et al. Climate change, allergy and asthma, and the role of tropical forests. World Allergy Organ J 2017;10:1–8.
37. Ayres JG, Forsberg B, Annesi-Maesano I, et al. Climate change and respiratory disease: European respiratory society position statement. Eur Respir J 2009;34: 295–302.
38. D'Amato G, Pawankar R, Vitale C, et al. Climate change and air pollution: effects on respiratory allergy. Allergy Asthma Immunol Res 2016;8:391–5.
39. Krishna MT, Mahesh PA, Vedanthan P, et al. An appraisal of allergic disorders in India and an urgent call for action. World Allergy Organ J 2020;13:100446.
40. Anenberg SC, Henze DK, Tinney V, et al. Estimates of the global burden of ambient PM2.5, ozone, and NO2 on asthma incidence and emergency room visits. Environ Health Perspect 2018;126:107004.
41. Rogers CA, Wayne PM, Macklin EA, et al. Interaction of the onset of spring and elevated atmospheric CO2 on ragweed (Ambrosia artemisiifolia L.) pollen production. Environ Health Perspect 2006;114:865–9.
42. Kaushik G, Khalid MA. Climate change impact on forestry in India. In: Lichtfouse E, editor. Alternative farming systems, biotechnology, drought stress and ecological fertilisation. Sustainable agriculture reviews. Dordrecht (the Netherlands): Springer; 2011.
43. Ziska LH, Beggs PJ. Anthropogenic climate change and allergen exposure: the role of plant biology. J Allergy Clin Immunol 2012;129:27–32.
44. National Research Council, NRC. Managing water resources in the west under conditions of climate uncertainty: a proceedings. Washington, DC: The National Academies Press; 1991.
45. Jagadish SVK, Bahuguna RN, Djanaguiraman M, et al. Implications of high temperature and elevated CO2 on flowering time in plants. Front Plant Sci 2016; 7:913.
46. Shivanna KR, Tandon R. Reproductive ecology of flowering plants: a manual. New Delhi (India): Springer; 2014. p. 107–23.
47. Primack RB, Higuchi H, Miller-Rushing AJ. The impact of climate change on cherry trees and other species in Japan. Biol Conserv 2009;142:1943–9.
48. Menzel A. Trends in phenological phases in Europe between 1951 and 1996. Int J Biometeorol 2000;44:76–81.
49. Crimmins T, Crimmins M, Bertelsen CD. Onset of summer flowering in a 'Sky Island' is driven by monsoon moisture. New Phytol 2011;191:468–79.
50. Hulme PE. Contrasting impacts of climate-driven flowering phenology on changes in alien and native plant species distributions. New Phytol 2011;89: 272–81.
51. Rana JC, Sharma SK. Plant genetic resources management under emerging climate change. Indian J Genet 2009;69:267–83.
52. Intergovernmental Panel on Climate Change, IPCC. In: Callander BA, Varney SK, editors. Climate Change 1992. The supplementary report to the IPCC scientific assessment. Houghton GT. Cambridge (United Kingdom): Cambridge University Press; 1992.
53. Blando J, Bielory L, Nguyen V, et al. Anthropogenic climate change and allergic diseases. Atmosphere 2012;3:200–12.
54. Singh AB, Mathur C. An aerobiological perspective in allergy and asthma. Asia Pac Allergy 2012;2:210–22.

55. Jarzen DM, Nichols DJ. Pollen. In: Jansonius J, McGregor DC, editors. Paly-nology: principles and applications. The University of California, American Association of Stratigraphic Palynologist Foundation; 1996. p. 261–91.

56. Stephen A. Pollen – a microscopic wonder of plant kingdom. Int J Adv Res Biol Sci 2014;1:45–62.

57. Kremp OW. Morphologic encyclopedia of palynology. Tucson (AZ): University of Arizona Press; 1965. p. 263.

58. Agashe SN. Pollen morphology. In: pollen and spores: applications with special emphasis on aerobiology and allergy. Boca Raton: CRC Press; 2019.

59. Koenig JQ, Morgan MS, Horike M, et al. The effect of sulfur dioxide on nasal and lung function in adolescents with extrinsic asthma. J Allergy Clin Immunol 1985; 76:813–8.

60. Molfino NA, Wright SC, Katz I, et al. Effect of low concentrations of ozone on inhaled allergen responses in asthmatic subjects. Lancet 1991;338:199–203.

61. Rusznak C, Devalia JL, Davies RJ. The airway response to asthmatics to inhaled allergen after exposure to pollutants. Thorax 1996;51:1105–8.

62. Puttonen E, Pilstrom L. Purification of birch pollen extract by gel filtration. Chemical and immunological characterization of the fractions. Int Arch Allergy Appl Immunol 1980;61:299–307.

63. Richman PG, Gissel DS. A procedure for total protein determination with special application to allergenic extract standardization. J Biol Stand 1988;16:225–38.

64. Park JW, Ko SH, Kim CW, et al. Identification and characterization of the major allergen of the *Humulus japonicus* pollen. Clin Exp Allergy 1999;29:1080–6.

65. Rawat A, Singh A, Singh AB, et al. Clinical and immunologic evaluation of Cedrus deodara pollen: a new allergen from India. Allergy 2000;55:620–6.

66. O'Conner CJ, Ashford KP, Speeding DJ. Germination and metabolism of *Pinus radiata* pollen in the presence of sulfur dioxide. J Plant Physiol 1987;126:373–8.

67. Omura M, Matsuta N, Mariguchi T, et al. Variation in physiological and genetic characteristics and pollen grain number in Japanese pear depending on the growing conditions. Bull Fruit Tree Res 1989;16:11–24.

68. Majd A, Ghanati F. The effect of air pollution on the allergenicity of Pinus elderica (Pinaceae) pollen. Grana 1995;34:208–11.

69. Ruffin J, Liu MYG, Sessoms R, et al. Effects of certain atmospheric pollutants (SO, NO and CO) on the soluble amino acids, molecular weight and antigenicity of some airborne pollen grains. Cytobios 1986;46:119–29.

70. Bist A, Pandit T, Bhatnagar AK. Variability in protein content of pollen of Castor bean (*Ricinus communis*) before and after exposure to the air pollutants SO and NO. Grana 2004;43:94–100.

71. Kalkar SA, Jaiswal R. Effects of industrial pollution on pollen morphology of Cassia species. Int J Life Sci 2014;2:17–22.

72. Talukdar P, Dutta A. Biomonitoring with special reference to leaf and pollen morphology in Cassia sophera L. to detect roadside air pollution. World Scientific News 2018;105:168–81.

73. Hinge V, Tidke J, Das B, et al. Air pollution exacerbates effect of allergenic pollen proteins of *Cassia siamea*: a preliminary report. Grana 2017;56:147–54.

74. Dahl A, van den Bosch M, Ogren T. Allergic pollen emissions from vegetation-threats and prevention. In: van den Bosch M, Bird W, editors. Oxford textbook of nature and public health: the role of nature in improving the health of a population. Oxford Textbooks in Public Health. United Kingdom: Oxford University Press; 2018.

75. Oh JW. Pollen and climate. In pollen allergy in a changing world . A guide to sci-entific understanding and clinical practice. Singapore: SpringerNature; 2018.
76. Park HJ, Lee JH, Park KH, et al. A six-year study on the changes in airborne pol-len counts and skin positivity rates in Korea: 2008–2013. Yonsei Med J 2016;57: 714–20.
77. Sedghy F, Varasteh AR, Sankian M, et al. Interaction between air pollutants and pollen grains: the role on the rising trend in allergy. Rep Biochem Mol Biol 2018; 6:219–24.
78. iron N, Nepi M, Pacini E. Water status and associated processes mark critical stages in pollen development and functioning. Ann Bot 2012;109:1201–14.
79. Ciampolini F, Shivanna KR, Cresti M. High humidity and heat stress causes dissociation of endoplasmic reticulum in tobacco plants. Plant Biol 1990;104: 110–6.
80. Singh AB, Babu CR. Studies on pollen allergy in Delhi: diurnal periodicity of common allergenic pollen. Allergy 1980;35:311–7.
81. Jagadish SVK, Muthurajan R, Oane R, et al. Physiological and proteomic ap-proaches to address heat tolerance during anthesis in rice (Oryza sativa L.). J Exp Bot 2010;61:143e156.
82. Cunningham DD. Microscopic examination of air. Calcutta (West Bengal): Govt printer; 1873. p. 58.
83. Shivpuri DN, Singh AB, Babu CR. New allergenic pollens of Delhi state, India and their clinical significance. Ann Allergy 1979;42:49–52.
84. Anonymous. All India coordinated project on aeroallergens and human health. Report. New Delhi (India): Ministry of Environment and Forests; 2000.
85. Singh K, Shivpuri DN. Studies in yet unknown allergenic pollens of Delhi state, metropolitan: botanical aspects. Indian J Med Res 1971;59:1397–410.
86. Malik P, Singh AB, Babu CR, et al. Atmospheric concentration of pollen grains at human height. Grana 1990;30:129–35.
87. Mittre V, Khandelwal A. Airborne pollen grains and fungal spores at Lucknow during 1969-1970. Palaeobotanist 1973;22:177–85.
88. Chanda S, Sarkar PK. Pollen grains as a causative agent of respiratory allergy with reference to aeropalynology of greater calcutta. Trans Bose Res Inst 1972; 35:61–7.
89. Singh AB, Kumar P. Aerial pollen diversity in India and their clinical significance in allergic diseases. Indian J Clin Biochem 2004;19:190–201.
90. Singh N, Devi KK. Aerobiology and allergic human diseases in Manipur. II. Airborne pollen grains of Imphal, Imphal District. Ind J Aerobiol 1992;49–60. Special volume.
91. Prado N, De Linares C, Sanz ML, et al. Pollensomes as natural vehicles for pol-len allergens. J Immunol 2015;195:445–9.
92. Sharma D, Dutta BK, Singh AB. Seasonal variation in atmospheric pollen con-centration in humid tropical climate of South Assam, India. Ind J Aerobiol 2010;23:28–37.
93. D'amato G, Vitale C, De Martino A, et al. Effects on asthma and respiratory al-lergy of Climate change and air pollution. Multidiscip Respir Med 2015;10:1–8.
94. Rong J, Michalska S, Subramani S, et al. Deep learning for pollen allergy surveil-lance from twitter in Australia. BMC Med Inform Decis Mak 2019;19:208.
95. Jalbert I, Golebiowski B. Environmental aeroallergens and allergic rhino-conjunctivitis. Curr Opin Allergy Clin Immunol 2015;15:476–81.
96. Beggs PJ, Katelaris CH, Medek D, et al. Differences in grass pollen allergen exposure across Australia. Aust N Z J Public Health 2015;39:51–5.

97. Singh AB, Pandit T, Dahiya P. Changes in airborne pollen concentrations in Delhi, India. Grana 2003;42:168–77.

98. Davies JM, Beggs PJ, Medek DE, et al. Trans-disciplinary research in synthesis of grass pollen aerobiology and its importance for respiratory health in Australasia. Sci Total Environ 2015;534:85–96.

99. D'Amato G, Tedeschini E, Frenguelli G, et al. Allergens as trigger factors for allergic respiratory diseases and severe asthma during thunderstorms in pollen season. Aerobiologia 2019;35:379–82.

100. Weber RW. Meteorologic variables in aerobiology. Immunol Allergy Clin N Am 2003;23:411–22.

101. Packe GE, Ayres J. Asthma outbreak during a thunderstorm. Lancet 1985;326: 199–204.

102. Bazzaz FA. Ecophysiology of *Ambrosia artemisiifolia*: a successional dominant. Ecology 1974;55:112–9.

103. Sikoparija B, Skjøth CA, Celenk S, et al. Spatial and temporal variations in airborne Ambrosia pollen in Europe. Aerobiologia 2017;33:181–9.

104. Beggs PJ. Impacts of climate change on aeroallergens: past and future. Clin Exp Allergy 2004;34:1507–13.

105. Ong EK, Singh MB, Knox RB. Seasonal distribution of pollen in the atmosphere of Melbourne: an airborne pollen calendar. Aerobiologia 1995;11:51–5.

106. Calderón-Ezquerro MC, Guerrero-Guerra C, Martínez-López B, et al. First airborne pollen calendar for Mexico City and its relationship with bioclimatic factors. Aerobiologia 2016;32:225–44.

107. Werchan M, Werchan B, Bergmann KC. German pollen calendar 4.0–update based on 2011–2016 pollen data. Allergo J Int 2018;27:69–71.

108. Mandal J, Chakraborty P, Roy I. Prevalence of allergenic pollen grains in the aerosol of the city of Calcutta, India – a two year perspective study. Aerobiologia 2008;24:151–64.

109. Mari Bhat M, Rajasab AH. Flowering calendar of potentially allergenic pollen producing plants of Gulbarga. Ind J Aerobiol 1992;15:89–93.

110. Singh AB, Dahiya P. Aerobiological researches on pollen and fungi in India during the last fifty years. Indian J Allergy Asthma Immunol 2008;22:27–38.

111. Mondal AK, Mondal S, Mandal S. Pollen production in some plant taxa with a supposed role in allergy in Eastern India. Aerobiologia 1998;14:397.

112. Singh AB, Kumar P. Common environmental allergens causing respiratory allergy in India. Indian J Pediatr 2002;69:245–50.

113. Singh BP, Singh AB, Gangal SV. Pollen Calendars of different states of India. Delhi (India):CSIR Centre for Biochemicals, Delhi,India; 199.

114. Singh AB, Khandelwal A. An atlas of allergenically significant plants of India. Himalaya Publishing House; 2016.

115. KimS, Park H, JangJ. Impact of meteorological variation on hospital visits of patients with tree pollen allergy. BMC Public Health 2011;11:890.

116. Lee J, Lee KH, Lee HS, et al. Japanese Cedar (Cryptomeria japonica) Pollinosis in Jeju, Korea: Is It Increasing? Allergy Asthma Immunol Res 2015;7:295-300.

117. Yamada T, Saito H, Fujieda S. Present state of Japanese cedar pollinosis: the national affliction. J Allergy Clin Immunol 2014;133:632-9.

Climate Change and Extreme Weather Events in Australia
Impact on Allergic Diseases

Constance H. Katelaris, MBBS, PhD, FRACP[a,b,*]

KEYWORDS

- Australian climate • Extreme weather events • Respiratory health effects
- Aeroallergens

KEY POINTS

- Climate change factors have resulted in increased extreme weather events on the Australian continent with significant impact on respiratory health in particular.
- Extreme bushfire events leading to dramatic smoke plumes and the resulting air pollution affect the health and well-being of thousands of people.
- The worst ever epidemic thunderstorm asthma event occurred in Melbourne, Australia in 2016 at the peak of the pollen season having catastrophic consequences, as emergency services were overwhelmed and several asthma deaths were recorded.
- Climate change factors will cause alterations in plant distribution, pollen and fungal exposure, necessitating careful, and longitudinal aerobiological studies in order to prepare for the changes in respiratory allergic diseases that may arise as a consequence of such changes.

INTRODUCTION

Changes in climate are affecting, and will continue to impact, various disease states. Allergic respiratory disorders such as allergic rhinoconjunctivitis and asthma are affected both directly and by the various consequences that result from climate change. There are 2 aspects of climate change affecting respiratory disorders that will be briefly explored in this paper: firstly, the consequences of extreme weather events and secondly, the change in distribution of airborne allergens that results from various climate change factors.

OUR CHANGING CLIMATE

Several climate change-related predictions and observations have been documented for the Australian continent by the Intergovernmental Panel on Climate Change,[1] the

[a] Immunology and Allergy, Western Sydney University; [b] Head of Unit, Campbelltown Hospital, Sydney, New South Wales, Australia
* Department of Medicine, Campbelltown Hospital, Therry Road, Campbelltown, New South Wales 2560, Australia.
E-mail address: Connie.Katelaris@health.nsw.gov.au

Immunol Allergy Clin N Am 41 (2021) 53–62
https://doi.org/10.1016/j.iac.2020.09.003
0889-8561/21/© 2020 Elsevier Inc. All rights reserved.

immunology.theclinics.com

most authoritative international body reporting on the science behind climate change and its various impacts and consequences, in conjunction with the The Commonwealth Scientific and Industrial Research Organisation (CSIRO) and Bureau of Meteorology who have also documented several scenarios. Global warming has directly affected Australians with extreme weather events such as drought, major bushfires, thunderstorms, cyclones, and flooding.[2] Australian average surface air temperature has increased by 0.9°C since 1910 and may increase by 1°C to 5°C by 2070. The years 2013 to 2014 were the warmest 2-year period in Australia's recorded history, with 2015 and 2016 not far behind.[3] In recent decades more extremely warm months have occurred than extremely cool ones. Many heat-related records have been broken in the last 7 years. Continued increases in mean and daily minimum and maximum temperatures are predicted throughout all regions with high confidence. Australian average rainfall has been increasing since the 1970s, mainly due to an increase in wet season rain in northern Australia. During the cooler months, rainfall has declined in the south-east and south-west of the continent. Extreme rain events are projected to become more intense.[3] Tropical cyclones are predicted to become less frequent but more intense (category 3–5), with a greater proportion of severe storms reaching further south.[3,4] In Southern Australia, time in drought is projected to increase with the occurrence of more extreme droughts in line with the decrease in rainfall in these regions.

Extreme weather events such as cycles of severe drought and damaging flooding experienced in Australia are attributed to the El Nino Southern Oscillation (ENSO), which is determined by the atmospheric circulation patterns over the Pacific Ocean. Two phases of ENSO are recognized; the EL Nino phase causes severe drought over the eastern parts of the continent, whereas the La Nina is associated with warmer surface waters in the Pacific Ocean resulting in extra atmospheric moisture and higher rainfall over much of the continent leading to flooding in vulnerable areas. Changes associated with global warming are predicted to intensify the oscillations, leading to cycles of more intense droughts and flooding events.

Southern and Eastern Australia will experience conditions conducive to more severe bushfires because of warming and drying of vegetation leading to greater availability of fuels, and this has already occurred with severe fires in 2009 (the Back Saturday fires in Victoria) leading to terrible loss of life and property and again in the summer of 2019 to 2020 in NSW, Victoria, ACT and South Australia with similarly severe losses.[5–7]

Weather events such as those described earlier have immediate consequences on many aspects of human health but the aftermath of drought, fires, and floods also threaten our well-being. By destruction of crops and infrastructure, food supplies are affected and infectious diseases become a threat. Persisting poor air quality has a major impact on respiratory and cardiovascular health.

IMPACT OF EXTREME WEATHER EVENTS ON ALLERGIC RESPIRATORY DISORDERS

For individuals with allergic disorders, there are particular health considerations around extreme weather events such as bushfires, thunderstorms, and flooding.

OCCURRENCE OF WILDFIRES

Weather conditions caused by climate change will increase the frequency of extreme bushfires around the world and this is particularly so in Australia where longer fire seasons, starting earlier in the spring and summer, are predicted to occur with increasing frequency. Research suggests that as global temperatures increase, these events will become more frequent leading to lower rainfall and creating a drier feedstock for extreme bushfires. In turn, bushfire smoke and the resulting air pollution affects the health and well-being of thousands of people.[8,9]

Bushfires have always been a part of the Australian landscape but as Australia's climate changes, one of the most significant and devastating consequences will be the occurrence of more frequent bushfires that are likely to be fiercer and difficult to control.[10] Large wildfires tend to occur during drought periods and in severe fire weather, driven by high temperatures, low relative humidity, and strong winds.[11]

Bushfire Smoke Composition

Landscape fire smoke is a complex and dynamic mix of energy, water vapor, gases, and aerosols. Many of the gaseous compounds are strong greenhouse gases and are toxic to humans. The public health impacts of air pollution, including landscape fire smoke, have become more clearly characterized over recent decades.[12–14] Large human populations including those distant from the fires, can be exposed to the resulting smoke pollution causing measurable increases in mortality and morbidity.[15–17]

Although smoke exposure might cause minor irritation of the eyes or throat in healthy people, it can precipitate severe breathing difficulty in a person with asthma or other respiratory disease. The health impacts of air pollution derived from wildfires are driven by various factors such as the chemical composition and concentrations of pollutants in the smoke plume and the intensity and duration of smoke exposure during an event and the extent to which individuals can protect themselves from that exposure.[12] Health impacts are also tied to the prevalence of risk factors in the population, such as cardiovascular[18] and lung diseases, diabetes,[19] older or younger age, and lower socioeconomic backgrounds. Smoke exposure is known to disproportionately affect people with lung diseases,[20] and the evidence concerning impacts on heart diseases is emerging.[21]

PM2.5 Exposure

The health effects best studied as a result of bushfire smoke exposure are those resulting from exposure to PM2.5.[12] These particles penetrate into the small airways causing inflammatory changes as well as having an effect on the immune system. People who have chronic lung conditions such as asthma, chronic obstructive pulmonary disease, and emphysema are most affected in these situations.[13] Other detrimental health effects of PM2.5 include promotion of inflammation and blood coagulation; impairment of the respiratory, cardiovascular, and autonomic nervous systems; and increased risk of genetic mutations.[12] Short-term exposure is probably not hazardous for healthy individuals but for those with respiratory disease including asthma it may provoke severe respiratory compromise. For those who suffer from chronic allergic rhinoconjunctivitis, further irritation of conjunctiva and nasal mucosa is inevitable.

As in other parts of the world, in South Eastern Australia, bushfire smoke exposure has been linked to increase in mortality.[22] When considering health impacts, there are no safe levels of PM2.5 so those with underlying respiratory disease are at risk regardless of whether the source is wildfire or controlled burning.

A long-term practice for mitigation of wildfires has been that of controlled burns to reduce the fuel load of a particular area at a time when it is safe to perform the controlled burn. Days with ideal weather conditions when temperatures are mild and there is no wind can be chosen for the activity; the at-risk population can be warned ahead of time to ensure use of preventative medications and "safe havens" may be created, either in a controlled environment or via the supply of protective respiratory equipment. Wild fires and controlled burns generally result in different smoke exposures to human populations. When wildfires occur, smoke and pollution are distributed over a very wide area, so large populations are affected.[12]

THUNDERSTORMS

On 21 November 2016 the worst ever epidemic thunderstorm asthma event occurred in Melbourne, Australia. It had catastrophic consequences, as ambulance services and emergency services were overwhelmed with calls for help. Hundreds of people presented to emergency departments throughout the city; 35 were admitted to intensive care units and 10 victims died. From previous thunderstorm events, several factors were identified that were prerequisites for such an event—particular types of thunderstorm activity with outflows, high aeroallergen exposure, and a susceptible population.[23] In Melbourne on that particular afternoon a powerful front hit Melbourne causing a sudden drop in temperature, an increase in humidity, and a concentration of particulate matter. This occurred at the height of the Melbourne pollen season when grass pollen (predominantly perennial rye grass) levels were extremely high. The timing coincided with the end of the working day, so many people were outdoors, traveling home.

Thunderstorm asthma events are not unusual in some parts of Australia particularly in the southern regions.[24] Previous studies had shown that fine starch granules, less than 2.5 μm, are released from rye grass pollen following wetting,[25,26] and with certain weather conditions, these are available to be inhaled deep into the lower airways. In susceptible, sensitized individuals such as those with seasonal allergic rhinitis and asthma this can precipitate a severe asthma attack.

CYCLONES, FLOODING, AND FUNGAL EXPOSURE

Flooding events have been the most common type of disaster globally and are expected to increase in intensity and in frequency due to increasing sea levels and more extreme rain events.[1] The numerous effects on short-term and long-term health resulting from flooding have been documented.[27] Respiratory effects are of our particular concern. Mold inhalation can cause or exacerbate asthma and other respiratory illnesses. Asbestos and other toxins such as lead and arsenic are often liberated by these events and require precautions. As expected, there was documented heavy fungal growth after the devastating flood in New Orleans in 2005 (Hurricane Katrina). This led to marked levels of indoor fungi, endotoxins, and fungal glucans all of which are associated with adverse respiratory health outcomes.[28]

The workers conducting remediation in mould-affected buildings are at particular risk, so require adequate respiratory protection to carry out remediation. Increased respiratory symptoms were demonstrated in workers associated with clean up after Hurricane Sandy in the United States in 2012.[29] Hurricane Maria in Puerto Rico in 2017 was also associated with increased reports of asthma and respiratory symptoms.

Cyclones and extremely heavy rain periods resulting in flooding are all too common occurrences in Australia. Tropical cyclones are intense weather systems that occur in tropical regions of the world, including around Northern Australia. They are deep low pressure systems with extreme winds, rainfall, and destructive waves that cause coastal hazards such as storm surges, flooding, and coastal erosion. Recent studies suggest that there has been an increase in the occurrence of high-intensity tropical cyclones globally offset partly by a decrease in the number of weaker tropical cyclones. The most intense tropical cyclones have increased their wind speeds in all ocean basins including the Pacific.

Tropical cyclones in the Australian region are influenced by several factors and in particular variations in the El Niño—Southern Oscillation. In general, more tropical cyclones cross the coast during La Niña years and fewer during El Niño years. Other important factors include changes in sea surface temperature and changes in deep convection.[3] The Bureau of Meteorology advises that the Australian region (90–160°E) has, on average, 13 cyclones a year. Half of these occur in the Indian Ocean, off Western Australia. However, tropical cyclone frequency in the Australian region varies considerably from year to year due to the influence of naturally occurring climate drivers.[3] Increased rainfall intensity from tropical cyclones is pertinent to Australia, since these storms have historically been associated with major flooding. In addition, increases in storm surges and extreme sea levels are very likely to occur in association with tropical cyclones under future climate change. This change is independent of changes in tropical cyclone intensity and is directly related to increases in global mean sea level due to global warming.

Australia has a significant history of devastating flooding events costing billions of dollars and causing long-lasting health impacts. Tropical cyclones are among the costliest natural disasters to regularly affect Australia. For instance, insured losses from Cyclone Debbie in Queensland exceeded $1 billion in 2017, making it the most expensive cyclone in the state's history. Cyclone Yasi 2011 destroyed almost 150 homes and a further 2275 homes sustained moderate damage and left another 650 uninhabitable when it crossed the far north Queensland coast.[30–32]

Fungal growth and exposure may also be an issue for many people after heavy rains, even those who have not been affected by floodwaters. It is also the scourge of many Australian homes year-round.[33] Fungi in damp buildings can trigger nasal congestion, sneezing, cough, wheezing, and respiratory infections. It can also worsen asthma and allergic conditions.[34] People most at risk from detrimental effects of fungal overgrowth and exposure include those with weakened immune systems; allergies; severe asthma; and chronic, obstructive, or allergic lung diseases, Understanding extreme weather hazards such as tropical cyclones and how they may change as the climate continues to warm is valuable for increasing Australia's preparedness and resilience to such events.

IMPACT OF INCREASING POLLUTION LEVELS

The generation of greenhouse gases by human activity contributes significantly to climate change. Pollutants such as ozone, nitrogen dioxide, and fine particulate matter are generated from motor vehicles and industrial processes. With increasing temperatures and longer periods of sunlight there will be more pronounced peaks in ozone concentration.[35] There is epidemiologic evidence linking the occurrence of asthma, asthma exacerbations, and hospital presentations as well as other allergic conditions with increasing air pollution.[36,37] Experimental studies have demonstrated that pollutants can induce development of numerous hallmarks of airway inflammation and can stimulate irritant receptors in the lung.[38] For certain pollutants, particularly ozone and PM2.5, adjuvant effects that may enhance the development of allergy to certain pollen have been observed.[39]

CHANGES IN AEROALLERGEN DISTRIBUTION AND ALLERGENICITY

Changing climatic conditions such as increasing atmospheric carbon dioxide (CO_2) concentrations and temperatures are causing shifts in the geographic distribution of certain plant species and changes in the length of pollen seasons globally.[40–42] There are several examples of this; the most significant one for respiratory allergy is the expansion of ragweed into areas in Central and Eastern Europe over the last 50 years.[43] A variety of changes in distribution have been documented for several trees including Birch[44] where forests are retreating to more northern latitudes and for grasses[45] and weeds.[46]

Several climate change factors have been linked to changes in aeroallergen concentration and potency. Temperature increases and elevation of CO_2 levels in the atmosphere have been associated with longer flowering periods for some allergenic plants, with some data suggesting increased pollen production and even an increase in the allergenicity of certain pollen. For ragweed, increasing CO_2 levels resulted in increasing levels of the major allergen Amb a1.[47–50]

Lengthening of the pollen season has been demonstrated in the United States and in Europe where long-term pollen counting records exist.[51] Zhang and colleagues[48] have described lengthening of the ragweed pollen season in North America, a change that is more pronounced in the northern locations such as regions in Canada. Others have noted an earlier start to the spring pollinating season.[51] By documenting the phenology of several flowering plant species, Fitter and Fitter[52] have described advancement in flowering seasons of many species in Britain. Ariano and colleagues[53] have demonstrated not only a lengthening of the pollen season but also increased total pollen load and an increase in pollen sensitization among the population in Italy.

Australia has one of the highest prevalence rates for both allergic rhinitis and asthma, so many people are likely to be affected by changes in aeroallergen distribution and potency. Studies in Australia have demonstrated relationships between grass pollen and fungal spore exposure and hospitalizations for asthma.[54,55]

Far less systematic study has been done in Australia to map changing plant distributions although efforts at mapping seasonal patterns of grass pollen distribution have commenced.[56] Methods that may be used to enhance our ability to issue pollen forecasts are also being examined.[57]

Many of the allergenic species in this country have been introduced from the Northern Hemisphere. Without natural predators they have become established in a new environment and have the capacity to induce sensitization and allergic symptoms. One example of this is the plant *Echium plantagineum*, which after it was introduced to the southern states of Australia as a garden ornamental in the mid-1800s, became prolific and overran pasture lands. Its allergenic potential has been demonstrated and its pollen contributes to seasonal allergy in the southern states.[58]

Ragweed has also been introduced and is slowly spreading in certain regions. Increasing CO_2 levels can be expected to alter the distribution of various grass species with higher CO_2 favoring C4 grasses over the C3 species. Nothing is known about how climatic factors will alter the distribution and flowering of native Australian species and indeed, very little is known about their allergenic potential. Furthermore, there is very little published material on the aerobiology of various allergenic fungi and even less about fungal distribution and changes over time yet there are known associations between fungal exposure and asthma presentations.[55]

These deficiencies highlight the great importance for funding systematic study of the aerobiology of the various disparate regions of the continent so that changes in pollen and spore levels and composition over time and with the changing climate may be tracked and mitigation strategies used where necessary. Prevalence of allergic disease is already high in Australia and if the present situation continues and in fact worsens, as is predicted, our medical workforce will be ill equipped to cope with the greater demand from patients suffering chronic allergic and respiratory conditions. There is an imperative to begin up-skilling and training our medical staff to meet the challenge of yet further increases in patients presenting with allergic and other respiratory disorders, an inevitable consequence of our changing climate.

Clinics Care Points

- Climate change factors are already affecting the lives of those with respiratory diseases.

- Early warning systems for bushfire smoke and high-pollution days need to be refined, and mitigating measures to effectively minimize these impacts for vulnerable people require further study.

- Plant distribution and pollen and fungal exposure will change as our climate is affected. Long-term funding commitments are required for adequate monitoring of these changes allowing for development of reliable predictive models.

DISCLOSURE

The author declares no conflicts of interest.

REFERENCES

1. IPCC. Climate change 2007: synthesis report. Geneva (Switzerland): IPCC; 2007.
2. Penny W, editor. Climate change in Australia. Technical report. Melbourne: CSIRO; 2015. https://doi.org/10.4225/08/58518c08c4ce8.
3. CSIRO and Bureau of Meteorology. Climate change in Australia: information for Australia's natural resource management regions: technical report. Australia: CSIRO and Bureau of Meteorology; 2015.
4. Reisinger ARL, Kitching F, Chiew L et al. Australasia. In: Climate change 2014: impacts, adaptation, and Vulnerability. Part B: regional aspects. Contribution of working Group II to the Fifth assessment report of the Intergovernmental Panel on climate change [Barros V.R., C.B. Field, D.J. Dokken, et al (eds)]. Cambridge University Press, Cambridge, United Kingdom and New York, NY, USA, 2014. pp. 1371-1438.
5. Climate Change in Australia. CSIRO Australian Government - Department of the Environment and Bureau of Meteorology. Copyright 2007-2016. Available at: https://www.climatechangeinaustralia.gov.au/en/. Accessed April 13, 2020.
6. IPCC. In: Pachauri RK, Meyer LA, editors. Climate change 2014: Synthesis report. Contribution of working Groups I, II and III to the Fifth assessment report of the Intergovernmental Panel on climate change. Geneva (Switzerland): IPCC; 2014.
7. Steffen W, Rice M, Hughes L, et al. The good, the bad and the ugly: Limiting temperature rise to 1.5°C. Climate Council of Australia Ltd; 2018.
8. Clarke H, Smith P, Pitman A. Regional signatures of future fire weather over Eastern Australia from Global Climate Models. Int J Wildland Fire 2011;20(4): 550–62.
9. Jolly WM, Cochrane MA, Freeborn PH, et al. Climate-induced variations in global wildfire danger from 1979 to 2013. Nat Commun 2015;6(1):7537.
10. Vardoulakis S, Jalaludin BB, Morgan GG, et al. Bushfire smoke: urgent need for a national health protection strategy. Med J Aust 2020;212(8):349–53.
11. Meyn A, White PS, Buhk C, et al. Environmental drivers of large, infrequent wildfires: the emerging conceptual model. Progr Phys Geogr 2007;31:287–312.

12. Williamson GJ, Bowman S, Price OF, et al. A transdisciplinary approach to understanding the health effects of wildfire and prescribed fire smoke regimes. Environ Res Lett 2016;11:125009.
13. Reid CE, Brauer M, Johnston FH, et al. Critical review of health impacts of wildfire smoke exposure Environ. Health Persp 2016;142:1334–43.
14. Reid CE, Jerrett M, Tager IB, et al. Differential respiratory health effects from the 2008 northern California wildfires: A spatiotemporal approach. Environ Res 2016; 150:227–35.
15. Henderson SB, Brauer M, MacNab YC, et al. Three measures of forest fire smoke exposure and their associations with respiratory and cardiovascular health outcomes in a population-based cohort. Environ Health Perspect 2011;119:1266–71.
16. Faustini A, Alessandrini ER, Pey J, et al. Short-term effects of particulate matter on mortality during forest fires in Southern Europe: results of the MED-PARTICLES Project. Occup Environ Med 2011;72:323–9.
17. Johnston FH, Webby RJ, Pilotto, et al. Vegetation fires, particulate air pollution and asthma: a panel study in the Australian monsoon tropics. Int J Environ Health Res 2006;16:391–404.
18. Pope CA, Brook RD, Burnett RT, et al. How is cardiovascular disease mortality risk affected by duration and intensity of fine particulate matter exposure? An integration of the epidemiologic evidence. Air Qual Atmosphere Health 2011;4:5–14.
19. Eze IC, Hemkens LG, Bucher HC, et al. Association between ambient air pollution and diabetes mellitus in Europe and North America: systematic review and meta-analysis. Environ Health Perspect 2015;123:381.
20. Henderson SB, Johnston FH. Measures of forest fire smoke exposure and their associations with respiratory health outcomes. Curr Opin Allergy Clin Immunol 2012;12:221–7.
21. Haikerwal A, Akram M, Del Monaco A, et al. Impact of fine particulate matter (PM2. 5) exposure during wildfires on cardiovascular health outcomes. J Am Heart Assoc 2015;4:e001653.
22. Johnston FH, Hanigan IC, Henderson SB, et al. Extreme air pollution events from bushfires and dust storms and their association with mortality in Sydney, Australia 1994-2007. Environ Res 2011;111:811–6.
23. Thien F, Beggs PJ, Csutoros D, et al. The Melbourne epidemic thunderstorm asthma event 2016:an investigation of environmental triggers, effect on health services, and patient risk factors. Lancet Planet Health 2018;2:e255.
24. Girgis ST, Marks GB, Downs SH, et al. Thunderstorm-associated asthma in an inland town in south-eastern Australia. Who is at risk? Eur Respir J 2000;16:3–8.
25. Knox RB. Grass pollen, thunderstorms and asthma. Clin Exp Allergy 1993;23:354–9.
26. Suphioglu C, Singh MB, Taylor P, et al. Mechanism of grass-pollen-induced asthma. Lancet 1992;339:569–72.
27. Alderman K, Turner LR, Tong S. Floods and Human health: A systematic review. Environ Int 2012;47:37–47.
28. Rao CY, Riggs MA, Chew GL, et al. Characterization of airborne molds, endotoxins, and glucans in homes in New Orleans after Hurricanes Katrina and Rita. Appl Environ Microbiol 2007;73:1630–4.
29. Gargano LM, Locke S, Jordan HT, et al. Lower respiratory symptoms associated with environmental and reconstruction exposures after hurricane Sandy. Disaster Med Public Health Prep 2018;12:697–702.
30. Carbone D, Hanson J. Top 10 worst floods in Australia. Aust Geographic; 2012. Available at: https://www.australiangeographic.com.au/topics/history-culture/

2012/03/floods-10-of-the-deadliest-in-australian-history/. Accessed May 12, 2020.

31. Devin LB, Purcell DL. Flooding in Australia Canberra. Australian Government Publishing Service; 1983 (Water 2000: consultants report no. 11) (Department of Resources and Energy).

32. Alderman K, Turner LR, Tong S. Assessment of the health impacts of the 2011 summer floods in Brisbane. Disaster Med Public Health Prep 2013;7(4):380–6.

33. Du W, FitzGerald GJ, Clark M, et al. Health impacts of floods. Prehosp Disaster Med 2010;25(3):265–72, 35.

34. Baxi S, Portnoy JM, Larenas-Linnemann D, et al. Exposure and Health Effects of Fungi on Humans. J Allergy Clin Immunol Pract 2016;4:396–404.

35. Kinney PL. Interactions of climate change, air pollution, and human health. Curr Environ Health Rep 2018;5:179–86.

36. Bernstein JA, Alexis N, Barnes C, et al. Health effects of air pollution. J Allergy Clin Immunol 2004;114:1116–23.

37. Romeo E, De Sario M, Forastiere F, et al. PM 10 exposure and asthma exacerbations in paediatric age: a meta-analysis of panel and time-series studies. Epidemiol Prev 2006;30:245–54.

38. Nel AE, Diaz-Sanchez D, Ng D, et al. Enhancement of allergic inflammation by the interaction between diesel exhaust particles and the immune system. J Allergy Clin Immunol 1998;102:539–54.

39. Okuyama Y, Matsumoto, Okochi H, et al. Adsorption of air pollutants on the grain surface of Japanese cedar pollen. Atmos Environ 2007;41(2):253–60.

40. Katelaris CH, Beggs PJ. Climate change: allergens and allergic diseases. Intern Med J 2018;48:129–34.

41. Katelaris CH. Impacts of climate change on allergic disease. In: Beggs PJ, editor. Impacts of climate change on allergens and allergic diseases. Cambridge: Cambridge University Press; 2016. p. 157–78.

42. Ziska LH, Beggs PJ. Anthropogenic climate change and allergen exposure: the role of plant biology. J Allergy Clin Immunol 2012;129:27–32.

43. Richter R, Berger UE, Dullinger S, et al. Spread of invasive ragweed: climate change, management and how to reduce costs. J Appl Ecol 2013;50:1422–30.

44. Zhang Y, Bielory L, Georgopoulos PG. Climate change effect on Betula (birch) and Quercus (oak) pollen seasons in the United States. Int J Biometeorol 2014; 58:909–19.

45. Albertine JM, Manning WJ, DaCosta M, et al. Projected carbon dioxide to increase grass pollen and allergen exposure despite higher ozone levels. PLoS One 2014;9:e111712.

46. Makra L, Matyasovsky I, Paldy A, et al. The influence of extreme high and low temperatures and precipitation totals on pollen seasons of Ambrosia, Poaceae and Populus in Szeged, Southern Hungary. Grana 2012;51:215–27.

47. Singer BD, Ziska LH, Frenz DA, et al. Increasing Amb a 1 content in common ragweed (Ambrosia artemisiifolia) pollen as a function of rising atmospheric CO_2 concentration. Funct Plant Biol 2005;32:667–70.

48. Zhang Y, Bielory L, Mi Z, et al. Allergenic pollen season variations in the past two decades under changing climate in the United States. Glob Chang Biol 2015;21: 1581–9.

49. Wayne P, Foster S, Connolly J, et al. Production of allergenic pollen by ragweed (Ambrosia artemisiifolia L.) is increased in CO_2-enriched atmospheres. Ann Allergy Asthma Immunol 2002;88:279–82.

50. Beggs PJ, editor. Impacts of climate change on allergens and allergic diseases. Cambridge: Cambridge University Press; 2016.
51. Ziska L, Knowlton K, Rogers C, et al. Recent warming by latitude associated with increased length of ragweed pollen season in central North America. Proc Natl Acad Sci U S A 2011;108:4248–51.
52. Fitter AH, Fitter RS. Rapid changes in flowering time in British plants. Science 2002;296:1689–91.
53. Ariano R, Canonica GW, Passalacqua G. Possible role of climate changes in variations in pollen seasons and allergic sensitizations during 27 years. Ann Allergy Asthma Immunol 2010;104:215–22.
54. Erbas B, Akram M, Dharmage SC, et al. The role of seasonal grass pollen on childhood asthma emergency department presentations. Clin Exp Allergy 2012;42:799–805.
55. Tham R, Dharmage SC, Taylor PE, et al. Outdoor fungi and child asthma health service attendances. Pediatr Allergy Immunol 2014;25:439–49.
56. Beggs PJ, Katelaris CH, Medek D, et al. Differences in grass pollen allergen exposure across Australia. Aust N Z J Public Health 2015;39:51–5.
57. Devadas R, Huete AR, Vicendese D, et al. Dynamic ecological observations from satellites inform aerobiology of allergenic grass pollen. Sci Total Environ 2018; 633:441–51.
58. Katelaris C, Baldo BA, Howden ME, et al. Investigation of the involvement of Echium plantagineum (Paterson's curse) in seasonal allergy. IgE antibodies to Echium and other weed pollen. Allergy 1982;37:21–8.

Climate Change, Air Pollution, and Biodiversity in Asia Pacific and Impact on Respiratory Allergies

Ruby Pawankar, MD, PhD[a],*, Jiu-Yao Wang, MD, PhD[b]

KEYWORDS

- Climate change • Air pollution • Allergic disease • Asia-pacific

KEY POINTS

- Epidemiologic studies show that climate change, and indoor and outdoor air pollution affect respiratory health, including increase in the prevalence of asthma and allergic diseases.
- Asia-Pacific is the most populated region in the world, with a huge burden of both outdoor and indoor pollutants and household pollutants.
- Risk factors for the epidemic increase in allergic diseases in the Asia Pacific region are due to increased urbanization and environmental factors of air pollution and climate changes.
- Abatement of the main risk factors for respiratory diseases, in particular, indoor and outdoor air pollution, are needed to reduce the burden of respiratory allergies.

INTRODUCTION

Globally, there is an increase in allergic diseases with about 300 million people who suffer from asthma and 400 million from rhinitis.[1] Air pollution, climate change, and decreased biodiversity are major threats to human health with detrimental effects on a variety of chronic diseases in particular respiratory and cardiovascular diseases.[1,2] According to the World Health Organization, every year 3 million people die prematurely owing to outdoor air pollution; the heaviest burden occurs in the major cities of Asia, Africa, and Latin America.

Climate change is a result of global warming, and is often defined as the change of temperature and weather patterns over a long period of time. Epidemiologic and experimental studies have demonstrated the relationship between various

[a] Department of Pediatrics, Nippon Medical School, 1-1-5, Sendagi, Bunkyo-ku, Tokyo 113-8603, Japan; [b] Department of Pediatrics, Center for Allergy and Clinical Immunology Research (ACIR), College of Medicine, National Cheng Kung University Hospital, Tainan, Taiwan
* Corresponding author.
E-mail address: pawankar.ruby@gmail.com

Immunol Allergy Clin N Am 41 (2021) 63–71
https://doi.org/10.1016/j.iac.2020.09.008
0889-8561/21/© 2020 Elsevier Inc. All rights reserved.

immunology.theclinics.com

environmental factors and climate change on respiratory allergies.[1–10] However, the precise molecular mechanisms by which air pollutants and climatic change impacts allergic diseases are complex and not fully well defined.

Outdoor pollutants like carbon dioxide (CO_2), sulfur dioxide, ozone (O_3), and indoor pollutants like tobacco smoke and chemicals lead to limited plant, animal, and microbial life. This situation can then lead to immune dysfunction and impaired tolerance in humans.[7,8] Lifestyle changes such as a westernized life style, urbanization, and high levels of vehicular-induced pollution have been shown to correlate with the increased frequency of pollen-induced respiratory allergies in residents in urban areas versus with those in rural areas.[11] O_3 has been reported to cause respiratory symptoms by inducing increases in airway responsiveness, airway injury and inflammation, and systemic oxidative stress.[12] Pollen from high-traffic roads have a higher allergenicity and children living in closer proximity to heavy traffic roads have greater symptoms of respiratory allergies.

Weather changes, like wind patterns, precipitation timing and intensity, and global warming, may also have an effect on the intensity of air pollution. One of the effects of climate change and global warming that can threaten respiratory health is thunderstorms asthma, which can be fatal.[4,13,14] In fact, air pollutants can interact with allergen-carrying submicronic and paucimicronic particles derived from pollen or other part of the plants and these allergens can enter the peripheral airways inducing asthma in sensitized subjects.

Furthermore, changes in the environment and human activities have caused an alteration in the biodiversity.[1,15] Metagenomic and other studies of healthy and diseased individuals reveal that reduced biodiversity and alterations in the composition of the gut and skin microbiota are associated with various inflammatory conditions, including asthma and allergic diseases. Solid fuel derived from plant material (biomass) or coal for cooking, heating, or lighting are smoky, often used in an open fire or simple stove with incomplete combustion, and result in a large amount of indoor air pollution.

CLIMATE CHANGE AND ITS IMPACT ON POLLEN ALLERGENS

Climate change influences not only the levels and the type of air pollution, but also the levels of allergenic pollen. Global warming affects the onset, duration, and intensity of the pollen season, as well as the pollen allergen potency. Over the last decades, many studies have shown changes in the production, dispersion, and allergen content of pollen and spores, and that the nature of these changes may vary in different regions and species. Current knowledge on the worldwide effects of climate change on respiratory allergic diseases is provided by several studies on the relationship between asthma and environmental factors, like meteorologic variables, airborne allergens, and air pollution. Published data suggest an increasing effect of aeroallergens on allergic patients, leading to a greater likelihood of the development of an allergic respiratory disease in sensitized patients and an aggravation in patients who are symptomatic.[4,5] Ragweed pollen production was 61% higher per plant owing to a doubling of the atmospheric CO_2 concentration.[10] Furthermore, ragweed pollen from high-traffic roads had increased allergenicity owing to the pollutants. In Southeast Asia (eg, Taiwan), where perennial allergen exposure is most common the major sensitizing perennial allergen is house dust mite, cockroaches, and pollen in the context of a highly polluted environment[16]

CLIMATE CHANGE, AIR POLLUTION, AND RESPIRATORY ALLERGIES IN THE ASIA PACIFIC REGION

The global burden of ambient $PM_{2.5}$, O_3, and NO_2 on the incidence of asthma and asthma-related emergency room visits estimated in 2015 were 8% and 20% and 4% and 9% of the total annual global visits, respectively.[17] Anthropogenic emissions were responsible for approximately 37% and 73% of O_3 and $PM_{2.5}$ impacts, respectively.[18] Of all countries globally, India and China had the most estimated asthma emergency room visits attributable to total air pollution concentrations, respectively contributing 23% and 10% of global asthma emergency room visits estimated to be associated with O_3, 30% and 12% for $PM_{2.5}$, and 15% and 17% for NO_2.

Furthermore, 16 million new pediatric asthma cases could occur globally each year owing to anthropogenic $PM_{2.5}$ concentrations. The percentage of national pediatric asthma incidence attributable to anthropogenic $PM_{2.5}$ was estimated to be 57% in India, 51% in China, and more than 70% in Bangladesh. The estimated asthma incidence attributable to NO_2 and $PM_{2.5}$ translate to approximately 1:7 million disability-adjusted life-years among children (approximately 97% of these attributable to $PM_{2.5}$), adding approximately 8% to the most recently estimated disability-adjusted life-year burden from ambient air pollution across age groups. The atmospheric concentration of CO_2, the most important anthropogenic greenhouse gas, has increased from 280 ppm to 379 ppm in 2005.[1,2] About 75% of the anthropogenic CO_2 emissions to the atmosphere during the past 50 years resulted from fossil fuel burning.[18] The key determinants of greenhouse gas emissions are energy production, transportation, agriculture, food production, and waste management.[6] Moreover, rising temperatures contribute to the elevation of the concentrations of O_3 and PM at ground level.[9,10] Westernized diets and lifestyle and urbanization combined with increased vehicular emissions correlate with an increase in the incidence of respiratory allergies in people living in urban versus rural areas.[8,9,15] In South-East Asia, air pollution is a result of a massive migration of rural population from farm to city in recent years.

O_3 has been reported to cause respiratory symptoms by inducing increased airway responsiveness, airway injury and inflammation and systemic oxidative stress.[4,19] O_3 and fine PM 2.5 are associated with respiratory symptoms and increased use of rescue medication among asthmatic children using maintenance medication. A 50 parts per billion increase in 1-hour O_3 was associated with increased likelihood of wheeze (35%) and chest tightness (47%). The highest levels of O_3 (1-hour or 8-hour averages) were associated with increased shortness of breath and rescue medication use.

Particular PM and diesel exhaust particles, O_3, nitrogen dioxide, and sulfur dioxide can exacerbate airway inflammation in susceptible persons, causing increased permeability, easier penetration of allergens into the mucus membranes, and easier interaction with immune cells.[4] There is also evidence that predisposed persons have increased airway reactivity induced by air pollution and increased bronchial responsiveness to inhaled allergens.

Regional weather changes, such as changes in wind patterns, precipitation timing and intensity, and increasing temperatures, also affect the severity and frequency of air pollution. Tropospheric O_3, which is formed in the presence of high temperatures owing to the interaction between volatile organic compounds (VOCs) and nitrogen oxides, are increasing in most regions. From the study of the burden of air pollution and weather condition on daily respiratory deaths among older adults in Jinan, China, from 2011 to 2017, outdoor air pollution was significantly related to mortality from all respiratory diseases, especially from chronic airway disease.[20] An increase of 10 mg/m^3 or

10 parts per billion of $PM_{2.5}$, PM_{10}, sulfur dioxide, NO_2, and O_3 corresponds with increments in mortality caused by chronic airway disease of 0.243% at lag 1 day, 0.127% at lag 1 day, 0.603% at lag 3 day, 0.649% at lag 0 day and 0.944% at lag 1 day, respectively. The effects of air pollutants were usually greater in females. Sex, age, temperature, humidity, pressure, and wind speed were considered to modify the short-term effects of outdoor air pollution on mortality in Jinan. Compared with other pollutants, O_3 had a stronger effect on respiratory deaths among the elderly. In a study looking at the impact of air pollution on small airway dysfunction in China, a significant association was found between urbanization, cigarette smoking, passive smoking, biomass use, exposure to high concentrations of particulate matter ($PM_{2.5}$), a history of chronic cough in childhood, a history of childhood pneumonia or bronchitis, a parental history of respiratory diseases, and increase of body mass index by 5 kg/m^2, and small airways dysfunction.[21]

THUNDERSTORM ASTHMA

One of the effects of climate change and global warming is an increasing frequency and intensity of floods and cyclones.[9,10] An example of how this effect can threaten respiratory health is "Thunderstorm related asthma."[4,5,22,23] Actually, thunderstorms occurring during the pollen season have been observed to induce severe asthma attacks and also deaths in pollen-allergic patients.[22–24] Thunderstorm asthma refers to an observed increase in acute bronchospasm cases after the occurrence of thunderstorms in the local vicinity. Evidence suggests that these thunderstorm asthma epidemics occurred only during the pollen season, with pollen-allergic patients at highest risk. Events have been reported from Europe, North America, the Middle East, and Australia.[22] Previously, the largest documented outbreak occurred in June 1994, when 640 patients attended London Emergency Departments within a 30-hour period. This event has been greatly surpassed by a recent thunderstorm event in Melbourne, Australia, on November 21 to 22, 2016, when more than 9900 patients presented to hospitals with asthma attacks[23–25] (**Fig. 1**). In excess of 2300 emergency calls were received, and despite valiant efforts of emergency services, 10 deaths have been attributed to this tragic crisis. A pilot questionnaire study of 344 patients who presented to the emergency departments in eastern Melbourne found that the majority of affected patients (57%) did not have a previous diagnosis of asthma, although most (51%) of these had symptoms suggestive of latent asthma; (ii) rhinitis was highly prevalent in 88% of subjects, with 71% of these being moderate to severe; (iii) 46% of cases were born outside Australia with a mean duration of 16.0 ± 11.9 years living in Australia; (iv) there was over-representation of non-Caucasian population, with 27% identifying ethnically as Asian (Chinese, Vietnamese, East or South-East Asian), and 16% as Indian (including subcontinental Sri Lankan, Pakistani, or Bangladeshi).[23] This over-representation of those born outside Australia (46%), and of Asian/Indian ethnicity (43%), is far in excess of that expected in the resident population. This finding has been confirmed in a subsequent analysis across the Melbourne population.[24]

NOVEL CORONAVIRUS DISEASE 2019, ALLERGIES, AND AIR POLLUTION

Since its first report in Wuhan, China, in December 2019, the novel coronavirus disease 2019 (COVID-19) pandemic has become a global public health problem. Previous studies have found that air pollution is a risk factor for respiratory infection by carrying micro-organisms and affecting the body's immunity. In a study in China addressing the relationship between ambient air pollutants and the infection caused by the severe acute respiratory syndrome coronavirus 2 showed that short-term

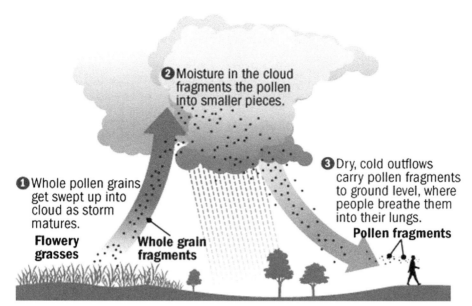

Fig. 1. Hypothesis for the mechanism of thunderstorm asthma. (*Adapted from* Department of Health and Human Services. Review of response to the thunderstorm asthma event of 21–22, 2016 Final Report. Victoria State Government 2017. Available at: https://www2.health. vic.gov.au/about/publications/researchandreports/thunderstorm-asthma-igem-review-final-report-april-2017 © Copyright State Government of Victoria.)

exposure to higher concentrations of $PM_{2.5}$, PM_{10}, CO, NO_2, and O_3 is associated with an increased risk of COVID-19 infection.[26] Patients with asthma and allergies are usually at greater risk of more severe outcomes with viral infections. However, recent reports have accumulated evidence that the prevalence of allergic diseases and asthma in patients with COVID-19 is lower than expected. Potentially, this finding is due to chronic and sustained type 2 immune inflammation in the lungs of asthmatic patients, or by the medications they use for asthma control, it seems asthma is not a major comorbidity and risk factors of the severe form of COVID-19.[27] Another potential factor could be the low levels of air pollution during the lockdown in many cities worldwide.

INDOOR AIR POLLUTION

Human activities, like the burning of fossil fuels like coal and oil, increase the amount of CO_2 that is emitted into the atmosphere, thus altering natural atmospheric greenhouse. One-third of the world's population uses solid fuel derived from plant material (biomass) or coal for cooking, heating, or lighting. These fuels are smoky, often used in an open fire or simple stove with incomplete combustion, and result in a large amount of household air pollution when smoke is poorly vented. Household air pollution accounts for about 3.5 to 4.0 million deaths every year. In Southeast Asia, many rural and even urban households use coal-based heating systems for cooking owing to financial reasons. Women and children living in severe poverty have the greatest exposures to household air pollution. Exposure to particulate emissions poses a variety of public health concerns worldwide, specifically in developing countries. One review summarized the documented studies on indoor PM emissions and their major health concerns in South Asia.[28] Alarming levels of indoor air pollution are reported in India, Pakistan, Nepal, and Bangladesh; Sri Lanka and Bhutan are confronted with relatively lower levels, although they are not safe, either. The reported levels of PM with a diameter of PM_{10} or less and $PM_{2.5}$ in Nepal, Pakistan, Bangladesh, and India were 2- to 65-fold, 3- to 30-fold, 4- to 22-fold, 2- to 28-fold, and 1- to 139-fold, 2- to 180-fold, 3- to 77-fold, and 1- to 40-fold higher than World Health Organization standards for indoor PM10 (50 $\mu g/m^3$) and $PM_{2.5}$ (25 $\mu g/m^3$), respectively. Regarding indoor air pollution-mediated health concerns, mortality rates and incidences of respiratory and nonrespiratory diseases were increasing with alarming rates, specifically in India, Pakistan, Nepal, and Bangladesh. A major cause might be the reliance of approximately 80% population on conventional biomass burning in the region.

VOCs are a group of carbon-based chemicals that easily evaporate at room temperature. Many common household materials and products, such as paints and cleaning products, give off VOCs. Common VOCs include acetone, benzene, ethylene glycol, formaldehyde, methylene chloride, perchloroethylene, toluene, and xylene. Several studies suggest that exposure to VOCs may make symptoms worse in people who have asthma or are particularly sensitive to chemicals. From a cohort study in Hong Kong regarding the household incense burning and children's respiratory health, incense burning was associated with 48.6 mL/min lower maximum mid-expiratory flow in boys.[29] In follow-up, incense burning was associated with reduced peak expiratory flow growth in all participants. These researchers also found that incense burning was associated with increased prevalence of bronchitis and bronchiolitis,

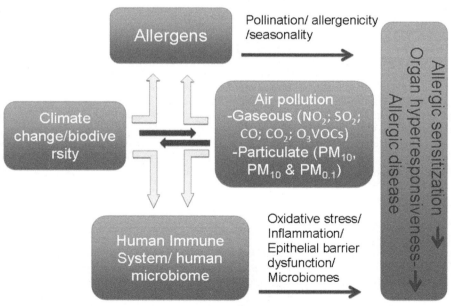

Fig. 2. Interactions of climate change and air pollution on respiratory allergies. (*From* Reinmuth-Selzle K, Kamp CJ, Kurt Lucas K,et al. Air Pollution and Climate Change Effects on Allergies in the Anthropocene: Abundance, Interaction, and Modification of Allergens and Adjuvants. Environ Sci Technol 2017; 51(8): 4119–4141 (https://pubs.acs.org/doi/10.1021/acs.est.6b04908); with permission.)

higher prevalence of pneumonia (odds ratio, 2.79) and wheezing (odds ratio, 1.49) in boys, but not in girls. The respiratory effects of secondhand smoke have been widely studied, supporting a causal relation between parental smoking and respiratory symptoms, including cough, phlegm, breathlessness, and wheeze, in children aged 5 to 16 years of age. From a cross-sectional study in Hong Kong on the relationship of exposure to secondhand smoke from neighbors and respiratory symptoms in never-smoking adolescents, they found in all study subjects that 33.2% were exposed to secondhand smoke at home, including 16.2% from inside the home only, 10.0% from neighbors only, and 7.0% from both. The prevalence of secondhand smoke exposure from neighbors was 17.1%, including 13.5% for 1 to 4 d/wk and 3.6% for 5 to 7 d/wk. In never-smokers (n = 50,762), respiratory symptoms were significantly associated with secondhand smoke exposure from neighbors with adjusted odds ratios of 1.29 for any exposure, 1.21 for 1 to 4 d/wk and 1.63 for 5 to 7 d/wk. Secondhand smoking exposure was associated with respiratory symptoms in never smokers. Country-wise data on the impact of air pollution on respiratory allergies in Asia-Pacific is summarized in the Asia Pacific Association of Allergy Asthma and Clinical Immunology White Paper on Climate Change and Air Pollution and impact on respiratory allergies of the.[30]

SUMMARY

Climate change has major health effects, including an increase in the prevalence of allergic respiratory diseases, exacerbations of chronic obstructive lung disease and premature mortality. These adverse health effects are seen especially in the most vulnerable like the elderly, children, and those from poor socioeconomic conditions. According to the World Health Organization, nearly 1.0 million of the 3.7 million people who died from ambient air pollution in 2012 lived in South-East Asia.[9] The Asia-Pacific has a huge burden of both outdoor and indoor pollutants, including $PM_{2.5}$, PM_{10}, suspended particulate matter, CO, O_3, NO_2, sulfur dioxide, NO, and household pollutants, including biomass and tobacco. Westernized diets and lifestyle, urbanization, air pollution, and climate change have contributed to through different interactions with the human immune system and allergens (**Fig. 2**)[31] and contribute to the increase in the incidence of respiratory allergies in people living in urban versus rural areas in the Asia Pacific region.

CLINICS CARE POINTS

- Patient's respiratory allergies like asthma and AR are well controlled.
- Adherance to medications should be checked.
- Digital/Mobile technologies to report patient status or patient symptom and medications records can be used to report the clinical status of patients.
- Advise patients regarding avoidance of exposure to air pollutants.

DISCLOSURE

The authors have nothing to disclose.

REFERENCES

1. Pawankar R, Canonica GW, Holgate ST, et al. WAO White book on allergy: update 2013. Milwaukee (WI): World Allergy Organization; 2013.

2. Haahtela T, Holgate S, Pawankar R, et al, WAO Special Committee on Climate Change and Biodiversity. The biodiversity hypothesis and allergic disease: World Allergy Organization position statement. World Allergy Organ J 2013;6:3.

3. Hegerl GC, Zwiers FW, Braconnot P, et al. Understanding and attributing climate change. In: Solomon S, Qin D, Manning M, et al, editors. Climate change 2007: the physical science basis. Contribution of the working group I to the fourth assessment report of the intergovernmental panel on climate change. Cambridge, (United Kingdom): Cambridge University Press; 2007. p. 663–746.

4. D'Amato G, Holgate ST, Pawankar R, et al. Meteorological conditions, climate change, new emerging factors, and asthma and related allergic disorders. A statement of the world allergy organization. World Allergy Organ J 2015;8:25.

5. D'Amato G, Vitale C, Lanza M, et al. Climate change, air pollution, and allergic respiratory diseases: an update. Curr Opin Allergy Clin Immunol 2016;16:434–40.

6. D'Amato G, Vitale C, De Martino A, et al. Effects on asthma and respiratory allergy of Climate change and air pollution. Multidiscip Respir Med 2015;10:39.

7. Pielke RA, Cecchi L, D'Amato G, et al. Climate, urban air pollution and respiratory allergy. In: Pielke RA, editor. Climate vulnerability: understanding and addressing threats to essential resources. Waltham (MA): Academic Press; 2013. p. 105–13.

8. D'Amato G, Bergmann KC, Cecchi L, et al. Climate change and air pollution: effects on pollen allergy and other allergic respiratory diseases. Allergo J Int 2014; 23:17–23.

9. Singer BD, Ziska LH, Frenz DA, et al. Increasing Amb a 1 content in common ragweed (Ambrosia artemisiifolia) pollen as a function of rising atmospheric CO2 concentration. Funct Plant Biol 2005;32:667–70.

10. Wayne P, Foster S, Connolly J, et al. Production of allergenic pollen by ragweed (Ambrosia artemisiifolia L.) is increased in CO2-enriched atmospheres. Ann Allergy Asthma Immunol 2002;88:279–82.

11. Whitmee S, Haines A, Beyrer C, et al. Safeguarding human health in the Anthropocene epoch: report of the Rockefeller foundation-lancet commission on planetary health. Lancet 2015;386:1973–2028.

12. Islam T, Gauderman WJ, Berhane K, et al. Relationship between air pollution, lung function and asthma in adolescents. Thorax 2007;62:957–63.

13. D'Amato G, Cecchi L, Bonini S, et al. Allergenic pollen and pollen allergy in Europe. Allergy 2007;62:976–90.

14. D'Amato G. Airborne paucimicronic allergen-carrying particles and seasonal respiratory allergy. Allergy 2001;56:1109–11.

15. Flandroy L, Poutahidis T, Berg G, et al. The impact of human activities and lifestyles on the interlinked microbiota and health of humans and of ecosystems. Sci Total Environ 2018;627:1018–38.

16. Liang KL, Su MC, Shiao JY, et al. Role of pollen allergy in Taiwanese patients with allergic rhinitis. J Formos Med Assoc 2010;109:879–85.

17. Anenberg SC, Henze DK, Tinney V, et al. Estimates of the global burden of ambient PM2.5, ozone, and NO2 on asthma incidence and emergency room visits. Environ Health Perspect 2018;126:107004.

18. D'Amato G, Pawankar R, Vitale C, et al. Climate change and air pollution: effects of respiratory allergy. Allergy Asthma Immunol Res 2016;8(5):391–5.

19. Baulig A, Garlatti M, Bonvallot V, et al. Involvement of reactive oxygen species in the metabolic path- ways triggered by diesel exhaust particles in human airway epithelial cells. Am J Physiol Lung Cell Mol Physiol 2003;285:L671–9.

20. Wang S, Li Y, Niu A, et al. The impact of outdoor air pollutants on outpatient visits for respiratory diseases during 2012–2016 in Jinan, China. Respir Res 2018; 19:246.
21. Xiao DW, Chen Z, Wu S, et al. Prevalence and risk factors of small airway dysfunction, and association with smoking, in China: findings from a national cross-sectional study. Lancet Respir Med 2020. https://doi.org/10.1016/S2213-2600(20)30155-7.
22. Davies JM. Pollen allergens. In: Nriagu JO, editor. Encyclopedia of environmental health. 2nd edition. Amsterdam (Netherlands): Elsevier; 2019.
23. Thien F, Beggs PJ, Csutoros D, et al. The Melbourne epidemic thunderstorm asthma event 2016: an investigation of environmental triggers, effect on health services, and patient risk factors. Lancet Planet Health 2018;2:e255–63.
24. Thien F. Thunderstorm asthma: potential danger but a unique opportunity. Asia Pac Allergy 2017;7:55–6.
25. Inspector-General for Emergency Management. Review of response to the thunderstorm asthma event of 21–22, 2016 Final Report. Australia: Department of Justice and Regulation. Victoria State Government; 2017.
26. Jiang Y, Wu X-J, Guan Y-J. Effect of ambient air pollutants and meteorological variables on COVID-19 incidence. Infect Control Hosp Epidemiol 2020;1–5. https://doi.org/10.1017/ice.2020.222, 2020.
27. Wang JY, Pawankar R, Tsai HJ, et al. COVID-19 and asthma, the good or the bad? Allergy 2020;00:1–3. https://doi.org/10.1111/all.14480. Available at:.
28. Junaid M, Syed JH, Abbasi NA, et al. Status of indoor air pollution (IAP) through particulate matter (PM) emissions and associated health concerns in South Asia. Chemosphere 2018;191:651–63.
29. Zhang Z, Tan L, Huss A, et al. Household incense burning and children's respiratory health: a cohort study in Hong Kong. Pediatr Pulmonol 2019;5484: 399–404. https://doi.org/10.1002/ppul.24251.
30. Pawankar R, Wang JY, Wang IJ, et al. Asia pacific association of allergy asthma and clinical immunology white paper 2020 on climate change, air pollution, and biodiversity in Asia-Pacific and impact on allergic diseases. Asia Pac Allergy 2020;10(1):e11.
31. Reinmuth-Selzle K, Kamp CJ, Kurt Lucas K, et al. Air pollution and climate change effects on allergies in the Anthropocene: abundance, interaction, and modification of allergens and adjuvants. Environ Sci Technol 2017;51:4119–41.

The Role of Extreme Weather and Climate-Related Events on Asthma Outcomes

Andrew Rorie, MD*, Jill A. Poole, MD

KEYWORDS

- Asthma • Thunderstorm asthma • Flooding • Hurricane • Drought • Wildfire • Mold
- Pollen

KEY POINTS

- Thunderstorms during pollen season have the potential to elicit asthma exacerbation epidemics.
- As prolonged heat waves and droughts become more frequent, the risk of large wildfires will likely increase resulting in poor air quality and worsening asthma control.
- A significant number of homes in the United States are currently affected by mold and dampness, which may aggravate existing asthma or provoke the development of asthma.
- Heavy rainfall events causing freshwater flooding, sea level rise, and increased tropical storm activity are likely to damage living structures and worsen indoor air quality.

INTRODUCTION

It has been well established that climate change is not only occurring but accelerating[1–4] The most significant driver of this change is raising atmospheric carbon dioxide (CO_2) concentration. Over the past 250 years there has undoubtedly been an increase in atmospheric CO_2 concentration and two-thirds of that increase has occurred within the past 50 years alone. There has also been a measurable increase in other greenhouse gases, methane and nitrous oxide, which have played an additive role.[2,5] The effects of these quantitative changes in greenhouse gases has been associated with witnessed glacier recession, artic ice thinning, sea levels rising, dispersal of plant and animal geographic range, longer and more abundant pollen seasons, and increased extreme weather events among others.[2,5] It has now been more than a decade since *Lancet* published their 2009 report on the health effects of climate change and stated "climate change is potentially the biggest global health threat in the 21st century."[1]

Department of Medicine, Division of Allergy and Immunology, University of Nebraska Medical Center, Omaha, 985990 Nebraska Medical Center, Omaha, NE 68198-5990, USA
* Corresponding author.
E-mail address: arorie@unmc.edu

Immunol Allergy Clin N Am 41 (2021) 73–84
https://doi.org/10.1016/j.iac.2020.09.009
0889-8561/21/© 2020 Elsevier Inc. All rights reserved.

immunology.theclinics.com

Climate change reflects any significant change in temperature, wind patterns, precipitation over extended periods of time, usually decades. Over the past several hundred years, there has been an observed 1°C temperature rise. The Paris Agreement has created a target to keep the increase well below 2°C to prevent the "tipping point," which could result in more catastrophic consequences. Ideally the goal would be less than 1.5°C, but to accomplish this it has been reported that global emissions would need to be reduced in half by 2030 and reach net-zero by 2050.[3,4,6] The purpose of this review is to draw attention to asthma-related outcomes attributed to extreme weather and climate change–related events to ultimately allow anticipation and planning for current and future needs with identification of vulnerable populations including those with asthma. There have been already more than 200 extreme weather and climate events since 1980 that have each been associated with greater than $200 billion in damages.[7] These events can include flooding rains, prolonged wet periods, prolonged heat waves, drought, wildfires, hurricanes, severe thunderstorms, tornadoes, storm surge, and coastal flooding.

The Global Initiative for Asthma (GINA) describes asthma as a heterogeneous disease associated with chronic inflammation and hyperresponsiveness of the airways. This is a common disease affecting up to 300 million people worldwide making it a global health problem. There is a rising prevalence in developing countries and rising treatment costs worldwide.[8] In the United States alone, asthma affects an estimated 26 million people.[8] Weather can affect airway hyperresponsiveness directly (eg, cold air) or indirectly by augmenting aeroallergen production and worsening air pollution. One of the hallmarks of asthma is variable airflow obstruction, which can be triggered by multiple factors: humid air, cold air, respiratory irritants (eg, smoke), aeroallergens (eg, pollens, dust mites, dander cockroach, and mold spores), exercise, infections and medications.[8,9] As the frequency and severity of extreme weather and climate-related events occur it will increase exposure to these exacerbating stimuli and directly impact asthma outcomes.

SEVERE THUNDERSTORMS AND TORNADOES

Thunderstorm asthma (TA) is a phenomenon of an observed increase in acute asthma attacks that occur following thunderstorms. Thunderstorm-related asthma attacks are associated with unusual weather occurrences with wind and torrential rain paired with high pollen counts. Although these occurrences are rare in the literature, they are likely underreported. A challenge to studying this phenomenon is tracking small, yet significant increases in asthma exacerbations following thunderstorms. An observational study of more than 215,000 asthma-related emergency department (ED) visits in Atlanta, Georgia, between 1993 and 2004 found an associated increase in emergency room (ER) visits on days with a thunderstorm ($P > .001$).[10] Although the study showed an increase in asthma exacerbations, it notably did not account for pollen levels or the time of year particular pollens would be expected present in an air sample. Between 1990 and 1994, Newson and colleagues[11,12] reported 38 occurrences with excess asthma-related hospital admissions and correlated 12 (38%) with thunderstorms. Similar descriptions of increased ED visits have also been reported in Canada, Australia, and England.[13–16]

There is no exact definition for TA and the precise mechanism remains debated. There appears to be an interaction when specific meteorologic and aerobiology factors mesh to produce a "perfect storm." One of the earliest observations was published in *Lancet* in 1983.[17] This report described a 10-fold increase in asthma exacerbations requiring hospital admission following a July 6 thunderstorm in Birmingham, UK. On that particular day, air pollution was low and pollen counts were high.[17] Since that episode there have been additional reports in the UK, Australia, Canada, Italy, Iran, United States, and Saudi Arabia of TA.[18] In many of these episodes there was such a spike in resources needed to treat asthma exacerbations that it overwhelmed the local health systems.

The most notable TA epidemic occurred in Melbourne, Australia, on November 21, 2016. This particular event followed a thunderstorm with high wind, torrential rain, and high pollen counts. Over the course of the evening and the following day, more than 8500 patients required treatment for asthma exacerbations and 10 deaths were reported. This rapid influx of patients with asthma severely stressed the local emergency services.[11,19] Similar reports of local health services being pushed to the limit occurred in England in 1994 during a TA event. At that time a sixfold increase in ER asthma visits was reported. More concerning was that 5 of 11 local emergency departments exhausted nebulizer face masks, 8 of 11 ran out of steroid tablets, 6 of 11 short-acting bronchodilator inhalers and 4 of 11 beta$_2$-agonist nebules.[20]

There continues to be debate about the mechanism of TA. The most agreed on explanation involves high levels of aeroallergens accumulating at ground level. These intact pollens are larger than 10 μm in diameter allowing them to reach the upper respiratory tract but are rarely capable of penetrating the bronchial regions. The most common appears to be grass pollen grains (30–40 μm) with additional evidence suggesting fungal spores may also be involved.[11,18,21] As thunderstorms develop warm updrafts of air rapidly ascend into the atmosphere. This air current pulls along the concentrated whole pollens until they reach the high humidity environment of the cloud base. Due to the wet conditions and through a process of osmotic rupture the pollen releases allergenic starch granules that are smaller than the 5 μm required reaching the lower airways. These allergens are then returned to ground level by storm downdrafts or potentially via rain droplets and released on evaporation.[22]

To date, grass pollen appears to have the most data to support it as the antigenic stimulus for bronchospasm in TA. Other pollen such as olive has been implicated in at least one episode of TA and fungal spores have been suspected in others.[19,23] There is, however, a strong association with grass pollen season and the reported episodes of TA in both the Northern and Southern hemispheres. Is this association simply because most thunderstorms tend to occur in late Spring and early Summer which happens to be grass pollen season or is there more of clear causative role of grass pollen? Marks and colleagues[24] reported a considerable increase in the concentration of ruptured grass pollen grains following a thunderstorm. This particular thunderstorm event resulted in increased asthma hospital admissions and was associated with a fourfold increase in intact grass pollen grains and a sevenfold increase in ruptured grass grains compared with 1 hour before the storm's outflow.[24] The ruptured grass pollens are capable of releasing large amounts of allergen-bearing starch granules. These particles were found to contain major grass pollen allergens and induced bronchospasm following bronchial challenge in sensitized patients.[25–27] Venables and colleagues[20] reported that before 1994 TA event grass pollen counts were at a 6-year high and mold spores were at a typical level. After the storm 16 patients who suffered asthma exacerbations were tested for specific IgE to grass pollen and mold mix by CAP (Pharmacia). Twelve of the patients had very high specific IgE to pollen (Class 4–6), and 3 had low or moderate IgE to mold (Class 1–2). Of the 16 patients, only 2 did not have specific IgE pollen, whereas 13 were negative to mold.[20] Marks and colleagues[24] proposed the following criteria for identification of TA outbreaks: (1) the occurrence of asthma outbreaks closely linked to thunderstorm outflows; (2) thunderstorm outflow events limited to late spring and summer when there are high levels of airborne grass pollen; (3) individuals with grass pollen allergy are most likely to be affected; (4) there is a close temporal association between the arrival of the thunderstorm outflow and a major rise in the concentration of intact and ruptured pollen grains.[24]

According to the National Oceanic and Atmospheric Administration (NOAA), there are an estimated 16 million thunderstorms worldwide each year and 100,000 in the United States. Approximately, 10% of these are considered to be severe thunderstorms, which must include hail 1 inch or larger, wind speed greater than 57.5 mph, or a tornado. As a result of anthropogenic climate change there has been an alteration of multiple environmental variables, which are predicted to cause an increase in the frequency and severity of severe thunderstorms throughout the United States, Europe, and Australia.[28–30] The most severe thunderstorms, those producing tornadoes, have also been affected by climate change. Although tornadoes can occur in all months, there has been a trend in the United States of "tornado season" occurring earlier each year.[30,31] There has also been an interesting trend dating back to the 1970s showing a decrease in the number of days per year with tornadoes but an increase in the days of "tornado outbreaks." These are defined as days with more than 30 tornadoes. In the 1950s and 1960s this was rarely reported, but by 2000 there was approximately 20 of these days and by the end of the decade the number had increased to nearly 60.[30,32]

Severe thunderstorms are the type most associated with TA and the projected increase in severe thunderstorm activity raises particular concern for widespread asthma outbreaks. A second requirement for TA appears to be high pollen counts, particularly grass pollen, and this too has been augmented by climate change. Grass pollen is one of the leading aeroallergens worldwide, as up to 20% of the land surface is covered by grassland.[33,34] There are multiple weather variables that influence pollen production including mean daily temperature, maximum temperature, minimum temperature, average wind speed, atmospheric CO_2, relative humidity, accumulated sunshine hours and rainfall.[21,35] There have been reports throughout the world (eg, United States, Canada, Poland, Italy) demonstrating increased duration of pollen season, peak pollen concentration, total season pollen load, and pollen allergenicity.[36–41]

HEAT WAVES, DROUGHTS, AND WILDFIRES

It is predicted that the world will continue to experience more frequent and warmer hot days/nights, more frequent and longer lasting heat waves, fewer days with frost, more heavy rain events with flooding, and paradoxically more periods of drought.[2,35] NOAA describes 3 different classes of drought: (1) meteorologic drought results from precipitation deficit, (2) agricultural drought due to soil moisture deficit, and (3) hydrological drought occurs from runoff deficit. The United States has experienced several significant droughts since 2011 in the Great Plains/Midwest and California.[42] Although there is no evidence to suggest global meteorologic drought trends, there are regions of the world where anthropometric climate change appears to be driving drought. It has been projected that future higher temperatures will likely contribute to increased drought frequency and magnitude in the continental United States.[42] These warmer temperatures paired with rising CO_2 levels will amplify pollen production to impact allergic diseases including asthma.[5]

Over the past several years, there have been serious wildfires throughout the world in Australia, Chile, and California among others.[35] Over the past few decades there has been a significant increase in wildfires in the western United States and Alaska.[43–45] Multiple factors are associated with the development of large wildfires including temperature, soil moisture, relative humidity and vegetation.[42] A large portion of the increase in wildfires in the western United States has been attributed to warmer and drier conditions and a clear link between drought and increased fire risk exists.[43–45] Wildfires can include forest fires, grass fires, bush fires and vegetation fires. These fires can be stoked naturally, accidently or implemented during deforestation practices.

Due to multiple climate driven factors a significant increase in wildfires is projected and years without extremely large wildfires will become extremely rare.[46,47] These changes will bring about an increase in natural air pollution with more fine particulate matter ($PM_{2.5}$), carbon monoxide (CO), polycyclic aromatic hydrocarbons, aldehyde, semi-volatile and volatile organic compounds.[48,49] The molecules have the capability of irritating the respiratory epithelium causing chronic inflammatory/oxidative stress, acute bronchospasm and subsequently asthma exacerbations.[50,51] Fine particulate matter has an aerodynamic diameter less than 2.5 µm allowing for deposition into lower airways. It is also a major component of wildfire smoke and has the ability to widely disperse up to 1000 miles away and last for several weeks.[52]

A severe and long-lasting wildfire occurred in Victoria, Australia in 2006 to 2007, and during that event there were 2047 emergency department encounters for asthma. Hikerwal and colleagues[53] reported an increase in asthma exacerbations with a positive association with wildfire-related $PM_{2.5}$. This association was found to be the strongest on the same day of smoke exposure and other lag day periods did not demonstrate a significant association. The strongest association for wildfire-related $PM_{2.5}$ and asthma-related ED visit was adult women.[53] Interestingly, there have been several reports of adult women being at increased risk for wildfire-related asthma exacerbation. A large southern California wildfire in 2003 resulted in an influx of cardiopulmonary associated hospital admissions. This wildfire produced a substantially large amount of smoke impairing air quality. During the fire the highest recorded 24-hour $PM_{2.5}$ was more than 240 µg/m^3. For comparison, the US National Ambient Air Quality Standard for 24-hour average $PM_{2.5}$ is 35 µg/m^3. During the period of wildfires, asthma admissions increased across all age groups by 4.8% (95% confidence interval [CI] 2.1%–7.6%) and a 26% increase in the period following the fires suggesting a delayed inflammatory response. During the wildfires there was an increased risk of asthma admission for female individuals ages 5 to 19 (49% $P<.02$) compared with male individuals and also women 20 to 64 years of age (41%, $P<.001$ compared with their male counterparts.[54] In June 2008, a lightning strike ignited a peatbog fire in North Carolina, and Rappold and colleagues[55] reported a significant increase in all asthma-related ED visits (odds ratio [OR] 1.65; CI 1.25–2.17). Another potential vulnerable asthma subgroup is obese children base upon observations from the 2003 southern California wildfires.[56] This study reported an increase in short-acting β2-agonist across all body mass index (BMI) groups, but the largest increase was in the obese (BMI >30) group ($P<.05$).[56] In addition, an 8-year study showed that poor air quality (>10 µg/m^3 increase in PM_{10}) was associated with a 5.02% increase in asthma admissions.[57]

Heat waves can be dangerous due to the physiologic stress that prolonged high temperatures can invoke and also their association with triggering wildfires.[58–62] An example is the 2010 prolonged heat wave in Moscow that triggered multiple wildfires in the forest and peat bogs surrounding the city. The estimated all-cause mortality for the heat wave of 2010 was approximately 55,000. Shaposhnikov and colleagues[60] reported excess mortality during this period in subjects with underlying respiratory disease (relative risk (RR): 2.05, CI 1.80 to 2.39). An extreme heat wave in Omaha, Nebraska occurred in 2012.[63] There were not any associated wildfires or unusually poor air quality associated with this event. Daily asthma admission was found to be higher during the heatwave compared to the same dates 1 year prior with more seasonable temperatures. The peak asthma admission rates coincided with the most consecutive days of intense heat and the apex was during the hottest time of day. Subjects who were children or African American were threefold more likely to be seen for an asthma exacerbation.[63] Kharin and colleagues[64] projected that heat waves that were historically once in a 20-year period will occur every 2 to 3 years throughout much of the United States by the second half of the century.

TROPICAL CYCLONES (HURRICANES/TYPHOONS), STORM SURGE, AND FRESHWATER FLOODING

Of the extreme weather and climate-related events, hurricanes are known to cause the most significant mortality.[7] The Intergovernmental Panel on Climate Change Fifth Assessment Report (IPCC AR5) consensus projects a global increase in tropical cyclone intensity, precipitation rates and frequency of very intense tropical cyclones. During the past century the global sea level rose by 8 inches in most areas of the world, which will aggravate storm surge from cyclones.[65] The US Midwest and Northeast have recently seen more flooding[42,65–67] and frequency of heavy downpours has increased globally.[68] The areas historically affected by flooding will also continue expand. The Federal Insurance and Mitigation Administration of the Federal Emergency Management Agency found that by the end of the twenty-first century the 1% annual chance floodplain area would increase in area by 30%.[69] The US Global Change Research Program has project with high confidence that the frequency and intensity of heavy precipitation events will continue to increase.[42]

Extreme precipitation can potentially damage buildings allowing for moisture to enter the living area. This provides an opportunity for mold growth and increased levels of other aeroallergens which can worsen air quality and may trigger asthma in sensitized individuals.[70] It has been estimated that up to 50% of homes in the United States have indoor dampness and/or mold. Home dampness can aggravate preexisting respiratory conditions and also may cause new onset asthma.[70,71] Targonski and colleagues[72] reported that multivariate analysis of asthma patients in Chicago, Illinois, were 2.16 times more likely to die when mold counts were greater than 1000 spores/m^3 compared with days with mold counts less than 1000 spores/m^3. There was a reported increase in asthma and asthma severity after the recent 2017 Hurricane Maria in Puerto Rico. The Associated Press attributed this to high mold counts, increased rodents/cockroaches in damaged dwellings and poor air quality associated with the use of diesel and/or gasoline powered generators.[38]

A review by the Institute of Medicine concluded that there was sufficient evidence of an association with a damp indoor environment and/or presence of mold and asthma.[35] A more recent report by the World Health Organization established a considerable number of childhood asthma is attributable to indoor dampness and mold.[70] Alternatively, removing mold and dampness from homes can improve asthma outcomes. This was demonstrated in a prospective, randomized, controlled trial of symptomatic asthmatic children where indoor mold and water damage was remediated in the experimental group. The follow-up period was 1 year and the remediation group had significantly fewer symptom days ($P = .003$) and fever asthma exacerbations ($P = .003$) as compared withto the non-remediation group.[73]

In 2005, New Orleans, Louisiana, was struck by 2 powerful storms, Hurricanes Katrina and Rita. These extreme weather events resulted in significant inland flooding and storm surge. Several post-hurricane studies reported heavy indoor fungi growth with high levels of mold spores, endotoxins, and fungal glucans.[74–76] Likewise, New Jersey was ravaged by Hurricane Irene in 2011 and Hurricane Sandy in 2012, which caused significant flooding and structural damage. Saporta and Hurst[77] reported that post-hurricane, patients had 34.6 times ($P = .0001$) more positive intradermal skin tests to molds than before the hurricanes, and 95% of patients tested had at least one mold sensitization compared with 62% ($P = .0001$) before the hurricane. In another study involving 3835 individuals surveyed who were involved in the reconstruction efforts post-Sandy, more than one-third (34.4%) reported worsening lower respiratory tract symptoms (wheeze, persistent cough, shortness of breath).[78]

Bangkok, Thailand, is located in a lowland area near the Chao Phraya River delta and is prone to flooding. In 2011, a severe flood, described as the worst flooding in Thailand history, lasted 175 days and killed 815 people. In addition to the loss of life there was considerable destruction to homes, including mold damage. After the floods, sensitization determined by skin prick testing showed a significant increase in *Alternaria* sensitization among children with asthma and allergic rhinitis.[79] The Hawaiian island of Kawaii was struck by class III/IV Hurricane Iniki in September 1992. In the post-Iniki period, physician visits for asthma significantly increased (RR 2.81; 95% CI 1.93–4.09) and asthma hospital admissions were 3 times higher.[80] As climate change continues to alter ocean levels, produce increased inland flooding from heavy precipitation, and coastal flooding from storm surge, indoor mold problems can be expected to worsen.[35]

CLINICAL CARE POINTS

- Thunderstorms during pollen season have the potential to elicit asthma exacerbation epidemics.[18] Staying indoors with the windows closed can prevent TA in sensitized patients.[35]

- As prolonged heat waves and droughts become more frequent, the risk of large wildfires will likely increase resulting in poor air quality and worsening asthma control.[46–48,50–52]

- A significant number of homes in the United States are currently affected by mold and dampness, which may aggravate existing asthma or provoke the development of asthma.[70,71] Mold remediation efforts can significantly improve asthma control.[75]

- Heavy rainfall events causing freshwater flooding, continued sea level rise and increased tropical storm activity are likely to damage living structures and worsen indoor air quality.[42,74–76] If working in an area with significant mold exposure wearing an elastomeric respirator is more effective at reducing exposure to endotoxins and mold than N95 respirators.[75]

Data from Refs.[18,35,42,46–48,50–52,70,71,74–76]

DISCUSSION

It should be recognized that climate change is not solely an environmental concern, but these changes are unmistakably interconnected to our health. The effects of climate change will significantly impact those with underlying allergic and asthma disease. Asthma is a heterogenous disease with multiple environmental factors that have been associated with pathogenesis, exacerbations and mortality. GINA estimates that up to 18% of the world's population has asthma making it a global health concern. As summarized here, high pollen burden linked with TA, robust indoor and outdoor mold spore levels associated with tropical storms, heavy precipitation events or poor air quality during wildfires attributed to drought conditions, impacts allergic and asthmatic diseases. To slow climate change it will take a united effort though all sectors of society. Interestingly, the long-term effect of the current unprecedented decline in carbon emissions and air pollution observed from intensive quarantine practices in response to the worldwide coronavirus pandemic of 2019 to 2020 is yet unknown.

In conclusion, the allergy and asthma community of scientists and clinicians should be proactive in research and clinical efforts to assure the safety and health of our patient population to include long-term and emergency preparedness resulting from climate-related events.

DISCLOSURE

J.A. Poole reports funding from the National Institutes of Health (ES019325) and National Institute for Occupational Safety and Health (U54OH010162); all unrelated to the present topic. A. Rorie has no relevant disclosures.

REFERENCES

1. Costello A, Abbas M, Allen A, et al. Managing the health effects of climate change: lancet and university college london institute for global health commission. Lancet 2009;373(9676):1693–733.
2. Stocker T. Climate change 2013 : the physical science basis : working group I contribution to the Fifth assessment report of the intergovernmental panel on climate change. , New York: Cambridge University Press; 2014. p. xi, 1535.
3. Watts N, Amann M, Arnell N, et al. The 2019 report of The Lancet Countdown on health and climate change: ensuring that the health of a child born today is not defined by a changing climate. Lancet 2019;394(10211):1836–78.
4. Tollefson J. IPCC says limiting global warming to 1.5 °C will require drastic action. Nature 2018;562(7726):172–3.
5. Katelaris CH, Beggs PJ. Climate change: allergens and allergic diseases. Intern Med J 2018;48(2):129–34.
6. Haustein K, Allen MR, Forster PM, et al. A real-time global warming index. Sci Rep 2017;7(1):15417.
7. Bell JE, Brown CL, Conlon K, et al. Changes in extreme events and the potential impacts on human health. J Air Waste Manag Assoc 2018;68(4):265–87.
8. Global Initiative for Asthma. and National Heart Lung and Blood Institute. Global initiative for asthma : global strategy for asthma management and prevention. 2014 revision. ed. Bethsda (MD): U.S. Dept. of Health and Human Services, Public Health Service; 2014. p. viii, 132.
9. Pennington E, Yaqoob ZJ, Al-Kindi SG, et al. Trends in asthma mortality in the United States: 1999 to 2015. Am J Respir Crit Care Med 2019;199(12):1575–7.
10. Grundstein A, Sarnat SE, Klein M, et al. Thunderstorm associated asthma in Atlanta, Georgia. Thorax 2008;63(7):659–60.
11. Dabrera G, Murray V, Emberlin J, et al. Thunderstorm asthma: an overview of the evidence base and implications for public health advice. QJM 2013;106(3):207–17.
12. Newson R, Strachan D, Archibald E, et al. Acute asthma epidemics, weather and pollen in England, 1987-1994. Eur Respir J 1998;11(3):694–701.

13. Bellomo R, Gigliotti P, Treloar A, et al. Two consecutive thunderstorm associated epidemics of asthma in the city of Melbourne. The possible role of rye grass pollen. Med J Aust 1992;156(12):834–7.
14. Celenza A, Fothergill J, Kupek E, et al. Thunderstorm associated asthma: a detailed analysis of environmental factors. BMJ 1996;312(7031):604–7.
15. Newson R, Strachan D, Archibald E, et al. Effect of thunderstorms and airborne grass pollen on the incidence of acute asthma in England, 1990-94. Thorax 1997;52(8):680–5.
16. Wardman AE, Stefani D, MacDonald JC. Thunderstorm-associated asthma or shortness of breath epidemic: a Canadian case report. Can Respir J 2002;9(4):267–70.
17. Packe GE, Ayres JG. Asthma outbreak during a thunderstorm. Lancet 1985;2(8448):199–204.
18. Harun NS, Lachapelle P, Douglass J. Thunderstorm-triggered asthma: what we know so far. J Asthma Allergy 2019;12:101–8.
19. Andrew E, Nehme Z, Bernard S, et al. Stormy weather: a retrospective analysis of demand for emergency medical services during epidemic thunderstorm asthma. BMJ 2017;359:j5636.
20. Venables KM, Allitt U, Collier CG, et al. Thunderstorm-related asthma–the epidemic of 24/25 June 1994. Clin Exp Allergy 1997;27(7):725–36.
21. D'Amato G, Annesi Maesano I, Molino A, et al. Thunderstorm-related asthma attacks. J Allergy Clin Immunol 2017;139(6):1786–7.
22. Taylor PE, Jonsson H. Thunderstorm asthma. Curr Allergy Asthma Rep 2004;4(5):409–13.
23. Pulimood TB, Corden JM, Bryden C, et al. Epidemic asthma and the role of the fungal mold Alternaria alternata. J Allergy Clin Immunol 2007;120(3):610–7.
24. Marks GB, Colquhoun JR, Girgis ST, et al. Thunderstorm outflows preceding epidemics of asthma during spring and summer. Thorax 2001;56(6):468–71.
25. Knox RB. Grass pollen, thunderstorms and asthma. Clin Exp Allergy 1993;23(5):354–9.
26. Suphioglu C, Singh MB, Taylor P, et al. Mechanism of grass-pollen-induced asthma. Lancet 1992;339(8793):569–72.
27. Yeh HC, Schum GM. Models of human lung airways and their application to inhaled particle deposition. Bull Math Biol 1980;42(3):461–80.
28. Radler, AG., P.Groenemeijer; Faust, E, et al. Frequency of severe thunderstorms across Europe expected to increase in the 21st century due to rising instability.NPJ Clim Atmos Sci 2019; Volume 2, Article number 30 [cited 2].
29. Diffenbaugh NS, Scherer M, Trapp RJ. Robust increases in severe thunderstorm environments in response to greenhouse forcing. Proc Natl Acad Sci U S A 2013;110(41):16361–6.
30. Kossin JH, Hall T, Knutson T, et al. Extreme storms. In: climate science special report: fourth national climate assessment. Washington, DC: US Global Change Research Program; 2017.
31. Tippett MK. Changing volatility of U.S. annual tornado reports. Geophys Res Lett 2014;41(19):6956–61.
32. Brooks HE, Carbin, March GW, et al. Increased variability of tornado occurrence in the United States. Science 2014;346(6207):349–52.
33. D'Amato G, Cecchi L, Bonini S, et al. Allergenic pollen and pollen allergy in Europe. Allergy 2007;62(9):976–90.
34. Garcia-Mozo H. Poaceae pollen as the leading aeroallergen worldwide: A review. Allergy 2017;72(12):1849–58.

35. D'Amato G, Holgate ST, Pawankar R, et al. Meteorological conditions, climate change, new emerging factors, and asthma and related allergic disorders. A statement of the World Allergy Organization. World Allergy Organ J 2015;8(1):25.

36. Ariano R, Canonica GW, Passalacqua G. Possible role of climate changes in variations in pollen seasons and allergic sensitizations during 27 years. Ann Allergy Asthma Immunol 2010;104(3):215–22.

37. Bogawski P, Grewling L, Nowak M, et al. Trends in atmospheric concentrations of weed pollen in the context of recent climate warming in Poznań (Western Poland). Int J Biometeorol 2014;58(8):1759–68.

38. Poole JA, Barnes CS, Demain JG, et al. Impact of weather and climate change with indoor and outdoor air quality in asthma: a work group report of the AAAAI environmental exposure and respiratory health committee. J Allergy Clin Immunol 2019;143(5):1702–10.

39. Zhang Y, Bielory L, Cai T, et al. Predicting onset and duration of airborne allergenic pollen season in the United States. Atmos Environ (1994) 2015;103: 297–306.

40. Zhang Y, Bielory L, Georgopoulos PG. Climate change effect on Betula (birch) and Quercus (oak) pollen seasons in the United States. Int J Biometeorol 2014; 58(5):909–19.

41. Ziska L, Knowlton K, Rogers C, et al. Recent warming by latitude associated with increased length of ragweed pollen season in central North America. Proc Natl Acad Sci U S A 2011;108(10):4248–51.

42. Wehner MA, Dokken DJ, Knutson T, et al. In: climate science special report: fourth national climate assessment. Washington, DC: US Global Research Program; 2017. p. 231–56.

43. Abatzoglou JT, Williams AP. Impact of anthropogenic climate change on wildfire across western US forests. Proc Natl Acad Sci U S A 2016;113(42):11770–5.

44. Higuera PE, Abatzoglou JT, Littell JS, et al. The changing strength and nature of fire-climate relationships in the northern rocky mountains, U.S.A., 1902-2008. PLoS One 2015;10(6):e0127563.

45. Running SW. Climate change. Is global warming causing more, larger wildfires? Science 2006;313(5789):927–8.

46. Stavros EN, Abatzoglou J, Mckenzie D, Larkin NK. Regional projections of the likelihood of very large wildland fires under a changing climate in the contiguous Western United States. Clim Change 2014;126(3–4):455–68.

47. Westerling AL, Turner MG, Smithwick EA, et al. Continued warming could transform Greater Yellowstone fire regimes by mid-21st century. Proc Natl Acad Sci U S A 2011;108(32):13165–70.

48. Kinney PL. Interactions of climate change, air pollution, and human health. Curr Environ Health Rep 2018;5(1):179–86.

49. Sapkota A, Symons JM, Kleissl J, et al. Impact of the 2002 Canadian forest fires on particulate matter air quality in Baltimore city. Environ Sci Technol 2005;39(1): 24–32.

50. Huang SK, Zhang Q, Qiu Z, et al. Mechanistic impact of outdoor air pollution on asthma and allergic diseases. J Thorac Dis 2015;7(1):23–33.

51. Kelly FJ, Fussell JC. Air pollution and airway disease. Clin Exp Allergy 2011;41(8): 1059–71.

52. Naeher LP, Brauer M, Lipsett M, et al. Woodsmoke health effects: a review. Inhal Toxicol 2007;19(1):67–106.

53. Haikerwal A, Akram M, Sim MR, et al. Fine particulate matter (PM2.5) exposure during a prolonged wildfire period and emergency department visits for asthma. Respirology 2016;21(1):88–94.

54. Delfino RJ, Becklake MR, Hanley JA. The relationship of urgent hospital admissions for respiratory illnesses to photochemical air pollution levels in Montreal. Environ Res 1994;67(1):1–19.

55. Rappold A, Stone S, Sascio W, et al. Peat Bog Wildfire Smoke Exposure in Rural North Carolina Is Associated with Cardiopulmonary Emergency Department Visits Assessed through Syndromic Surveillance. Environmental Health Perspectives 2011;119(10):1415–20.

56. Tse K, Chen L, Tse M, et al. Effect of catastrophic wildfires on asthmatic outcomes in obese children: breathing fire. Ann Allergy Asthma Immunol 2015;114(4): 308.e4.

57. Morgan G, Sheppeard V, Khalaj B, et al. Effects of bushfire smoke on daily mortality and hospital admissions in Sydney, Australia. Epidemiology 2010;21(1): 47–55.

58. Anderson GB, Bell ML. Heat waves in the United States: mortality risk during heat waves and effect modification by heat wave characteristics in 43 U.S. communities. Environ Health Perspect 2011;119(2):210–8.

59. Baccini M, Kosatsky T, Analitis A, et al. Impact of heat on mortality in 15 European cities: attributable deaths under different weather scenarios. J Epidemiol Community Health 2011;65(1):64–70.

60. Shaposhnikov D, Revich B, Bellander T, et al. Mortality related to air pollution with the moscow heat wave and wildfire of 2010. Epidemiology 2014;25(3):359–64.

61. Vandentorren S, Suzan F, Medina S, et al. Mortality in 13 French cities during the August 2003 heat wave. Am J Public Health 2004;94(9):1518–20.

62. Whitman S, Good G, Donoghue ER, et al. Mortality in Chicago attributed to the July 1995 heat wave. Am J Public Health 1997;87(9):1515–8.

63. Figgs LW. Emergency department asthma diagnosis risk associated with the 2012 heat wave and drought in Douglas County NE, USA. Heart Lung 2019; 48(3):250–7.

64. Kharin VV, Zwiers FW, Zhang X, et al. Changes in temperature and precipitation extremes in the CMIP5 ensemble. Clim Change 2013;119(2):345–57.

65. Melillo, Jermy MR, Richmond T, et al. Climate change impacts in the United States: the third national climate assessment. Washington, DC: US Global Change Research Program; 2014.

66. Mallakpour I, Villarini G. The changing nature of flooding across the central United States. Nat Clim Chang 2015;5(3):250–4.

67. Groisman PK, knight R, Karl T. Heavy precipitation and high streamflow in the contiguous United States: trends in the twentieth century. Boston, MA: Bulletin of the American Meteorological Society; 2001.

68. Kunkel KE, Karl TR, Brooks H, et al. Monitoring and understanding trends in extreme storms: state of knowledge. Bulletin of the American Meteorological Society 2013;94(4):499–514.

69. AECOM, the impact of climate change and population growth on the national flood insurance Program through 2100. 2013. p. 257. Available at: https://aecom.com/content/wp-content/uploads/2016/06/Climate_Change_Report_AECOM_2013-06-11.pdf.

70. Clark, NA, Ammann HM; Brunekreef, B; et al., Damp indoor spaces and health. 2004, Institute of medicine committee on damp indoor spaces and health: Washington, DC: National Academies Press (US); 2004.

71. Mendell MJ, Mirer AG, Cheung K, et al. Respiratory and allergic health effects of dampness, mold, and dampness-related agents: a review of the epidemiologic evidence. Environ Health Perspect 2011;119(6):748–56.
72. Targonski PV, Persky VW, Ramekrishnan V. Effect of environmental molds on risk of death from asthma during the pollen season. J Allergy Clin Immunol 1995;95(5 Pt 1):955–61.
73. Kercsmar CM, Dearborn DG, Schluchter M, et al. Reduction in asthma morbidity in children as a result of home remediation aimed at moisture sources. Environ Health Perspect 2006;114(10):1574–80.
74. Adhikari A, Jung J, Reponen T, et al. Aerosolization of fungi, (1–>3)-beta-D glucan, and endotoxin from flood-affected materials collected in New Orleans homes. Environ Res 2009;109(3):215–24.
75. Chew GL, Wilson J, Rabito FA, et al. Mold and endotoxin levels in the aftermath of Hurricane Katrina: a pilot project of homes in New Orleans undergoing renovation. Environ Health Perspect 2006;114(12):1883–9.
76. Rao CY, Riggs MA, Chew GL, et al. Characterization of airborne molds, endotoxins, and glucans in homes in New Orleans after Hurricanes Katrina and Rita. Appl Environ Microbiol 2007;73(5):1630–4.
77. Saporta D, Hurst D. Increased sensitization to mold and allergens measured by intradermal skin testing followig hurricanes. J Environ Public Health 2017;2017: 2793820.
78. Hurst LM, Locke S, Jordan HT, et al. Lower respiratory symptoms associated with environmental and reconstruction exposures after hurricane sandy. Disaster Med Public Health Prep 2018;12(6):697–702.
79. Visitsunthorn N, Chaimongkol W, Visitsunthorn K, et al. Great flood and aeroallergen sensitization in children with asthma and/or allergic rhinitis. Asian Pac J Allergy Immunol 2018;36(2):69–76.
80. Hendrickson LA, Vogt RL, Goebert D, et al. Morbidity on Kauai before and after Hurricane Iniki. Prev Med 1997;26(5 Pt 1):711–6.

Insect Migration and Changes in Venom Allergy due to Climate Change

Jeffrey G. Demain, MD[1]

KEYWORDS

- Insect • Hymenoptera • Climate Change • Bee • Anaphylaxis • Venom
- Distribution

KEY POINTS

- Temperature increase, as related to climate change, impacts the range and distribution of stinging insects.
- Expansion of stinging and urticating insects expanding toward the poles will increase potential for human contact, increased risk of envenomation and potential increased frequency of allergic reactions.
- Allergist/Immunologists should be aware of the changing environment as a result of climate warming.

INTRODUCTION

The evidence that climate change is occurring is overwhelming. Recent work on climate change has helped advance our understanding of the influence environmental changes have on insect dynamics regarding population and redistribution. Insects are ectothermic animals, whose physiologies are strongly influenced by variations in the microclimate, particularly temperature.[1] There are only a few large-scale studies specifically addressing insects as a bellwether of our changing climate. This review highlights some changes in insect behaviors, particularly those that impact allergy, correlated with the direct and indirect effects of climate change and shifts in seasons.

Global, annually averaged surface air temperature has increased by approximately 1.8°F (1.0°C) over the past 115 years (1901–2016) with annual average near-surface air temperatures across Alaska and the Arctic increasing more than twice as fast as the global average temperature.[2] Globally, this period is now the warmest in the history of modern civilization. This past decade has seen record-breaking, climate-related weather extremes, and the warmest years on record for the globe.[2] These trends

Department of Pediatrics, Allergy Asthma & Immunology Center of Alaska, University of Washington, Seattle, WA, USA
[1] Present address: 3841 Piper Street, Suite T4-054, Anchorage, AK 99508.
E-mail address: jdemain@allergyalaska.com

Immunol Allergy Clin N Am 41 (2021) 85–95
https://doi.org/10.1016/j.iac.2020.09.010
0889-8561/21/© 2020 Elsevier Inc. All rights reserved.
immunology.theclinics.com

are expected to continue over climate timescales. There are many indicators of climate change, particularly physical responses, such as changes in surface temperature, atmospheric water vapor, precipitation, severe weather events, retreating glaciers, sea level rise, and diminishing sea and land ice.[2,3]

Several factors can influence distribution of insects, climate change is but one of them. Species redistribution and biodiversity loss has been significantly impacted by urbanization. Other key elements of biodiversity include genetic diversity of species, the richness of local and global species, the spatial extent and the state of natural habitats, and the functioning of ecosystems.[4,5] Because of the many variables, it is difficult to dissect out the effects of climate change versus habitat change. Therefore, modeling based on current trends, using best and worst case scenarios with regard to insect redistribution, may not reflect the many other factors of biodiversity and may not reflect real world interactions.[6] Few studies have specifically addressed the direct impact of venomous insect redistribution on human health, instead focusing on recognized changes in patterns and projected response to changing climate variables.

HYMENOPTERA

Hymenoptera, the largest order of insects, account for more than 10 million stings in humans worldwide annually.[7] It is estimated that potentially life-threatening systemic reactions to Hymenoptera stings occur in 0.4% to 0.8% of children and 3% of adults.[8] Populations of Hymenoptera, such as *Vespula*, have extended their range in both the Northern and Southern Hemispheres. The adaptation skills of *Vespula vulgaris* enable it to live in a wide range of habitats, from very humid areas to artificial environments such as gardens and human structures.[9] Although some Hymenoptera species appear to extend range, others will likely lose range and decline.

YELLOWJACKETS (*VESPULA* SP)

Vespula germanica and *V vulgaris* are widespread in Europe and North America and have subsequently been introduced into the Southern Hemisphere. *V germanica* became established in New Zealand in 1945 and Australia in 1959 and have continued to extend their range. It is projected that their range will continue to expand with the warming climate and as human populations and trade continues to increase.[9] These species are scavengers and therefore flourish in urban environments, resulting in frequent human encounters.[10]

The first 2 reported deaths from insect-induced anaphylaxis in Alaska occurred 2006.[11] This was in a period in which organized outdoor sporting events were canceled because of high levels of stinging insects, predominantly yellowjackets, in Fairbanks, Alaska.[11,12] Demain and colleagues[13] undertook a retrospective study to assess increases in patients seeking medical care for sting reactions between 1999 and 2007, using the Alaska Medicaid database. which represents 132,000 lives. These data were applied to different climate variables. The results demonstrated increases in billings for insect reactions throughout each of the 6 epidemiologic regions of Alaska, with increasing incidence correlating with more northernly latitudes. The largest percentage increase was in the most northern region, with an increase of 626% from the average incidence of 16 per 100,000 per year during 1999 to 2001 to 119 per 100,000 per year during 2004 to 2006 (**Table 1**). In summary, there was a statistically significant increase in patients seeking medical care for sting-related events throughout the state, with 5 of the 6 regions experiencing at least a 6-degree Fahrenheit increase in winter temperature. It was surmised that milder winters provided greater survivability of overwintering queens. The expansion of northern range of

Table 1
Annual and winter temperature increases and changes in insect sting incidence among Medicaid-enrolled persons, Alaska

Region	Largest Community	Annual Temperature Increase[a]	Winter Temperature Increase[a]	1999–2001 Insect Sting Incidence[b]	2004–2006 Insect Sting Incidence[b]	Percent Change in Insect Sting Incidence (χ^2 for Trend, P-value)[c]
Northern	Barrow	3.8	6.1	16	119	626% (13, P<.001)
Southwest	Bethel	3.7	6.9	62	133	114% (8, P = .005)
Interior	Fairbanks	3.6	8.1	333	509	53% (28, P<.001)
Anchorage	Anchorage	3.4	7.2	276	405	47% (22, P<.001)
Southeast	Juneau	3.6	6.8	221	279	27% (22, P<.001)
Gulf	Kodiak	1.5	1.5	437	487	11% (0.1, P = .75)
Statewide		3.4	6.3	254	364	43% (54, P<.001)

[a] Annual and winter average temperature increase (°F) from 1950 to 2006 based on data for largest community.
[b] Incidence per 100,000 Medicaid-enrolled persons per year for entire region.
[c] χ^2 for trend and P-value calculation based on individual years from 1999 to 2006.
From Demain JG, Gessner BD, McLaughlin JB, et al. Increasing Insect Reactions in Alaska: Is this Related to Climate Change? Allergy Asthma Proc. May-Jun 2009;30(3):238-43; with permission.

Vespula does not appear to be unique to Alaska, but rather has been observed in other circumpolar regions. In 2004, a Canadian entomologist and associate curator of the Natural History Museum in Los Angeles confirmed yellowjacket (*Vespula rufa*) in the village of Arctic Bay, Nunavut, Canada, at 73° latitude.[14]

Barnes and colleagues,[15] working in Fairbanks, demonstrated that although freezing causes death in the common yellowjacket, *V vulgaris*, this species can "supercool" to temperatures below minus 16° Celsius without freezing. In their study, snow depths of as little as 60 cm provided enough insulation to allow the overwintering queens to survive in hibernacula, maintaining an average of minus 6.5° Celsius, while average air temperatures were minus 19.4° Celsius (with minima often below minus 30° Celsius). These data illustrate that snow depth could be an important factor in the annual population growth of yellowjackets and potentially other Hymenoptera. Lester and colleagues[16] studied long-term population dynamics of *V vulgaris* over 39 years in 4 sites in the United Kingdom and over 23 years of data from 6 sites in New Zealand. They found that warmer winter temperatures and warmer spring temperatures were associated with increased *V vulgaris* abundance, although increased rainfall was associated with decreased abundance. They concluded that these data have broad implications that climate warming will have a direct impact on the yellowjacket population dynamic.[16]

PAPER WASPS (*POLLISTE* SP)

The most common Hymenoptera in North America is the paper wasp, with the European paper wasp, *Polliste dominula,* one of the most dominant of all social wasps. The specific epithet *dominula* is a noun meaning "little mistress." Prominent in Europe and Asia, it has also been introduced to New Zealand, Australia, South Africa, South America, and North America. Since the mid-1980s, the population of *P dominula* has expanded to historically cooler regions, especially toward northern Europe. Climate change, specifically climate warming. is speculated to have raised temperatures of certain areas enough to allow *P dominula* to expand into more northern regions.[10,17]

HORNETS (*VESPA* SP)

There are few data specifically addressing hornets regarding the impact of climate change. There are 22 species within the genus *Vespa*. Based on modeling, it is predicted that the Yellow-legged hornet, *Vespa velutina,* will expand its range into northern Europe and throughout the United States, except along the East coast.[18] Nesting patterns are quite different from *Vespa crabo,* in that they are larger in size and can have much larger colonies, up to 15,000 to 30,000.[19] These data suggest a significant increase regional predominance of these hornets, likely resulting in more frequent human encounters.

HONEYBEES (*APIDAE* SP)

In the United States, there are more than 4000 species of native bees (Bee Pollination. US Department of Agriculture. Available at: https://www.fs.fed.us/wildflowers/pollinators/animals/bees.shtml. Accessed March 18,2020). Bee species have demonstrated a very mixed response to climate change and warming temperatures. Although some have expanded range, others have experienced a reduction in both range and population. The Africanized honeybee (*Apis mellifera scutellate*) was introduced to Brazil in the mid-1950s, quickly escaped, and ultimately hybridized with the domestic European honeybee (*Apis mellifera mellifera*), creating what is commonly termed the

"Africanized honeybee."[7] The venom from Africanized honeybees is essentially identical to their domestic cousins, as is the venom volume per sting.[20] However, unlike the single sting of a domestic honeybee, Africanized honeybees often swarm and sting in large numbers and pursue their victim for much longer distances. The domain of the Africanized honeybee in the United States was initially had limited distribution, predominantly Texas, New Mexico, Arizona, Nevada, and California.[7,8,11] However, by 2009, the Africanized honeybee had almost doubled its range, now in 10 states[8] (**Fig. 1**). Continued northward expansion of the Africanized honeybee is predicted, largely impacted by temperature warming. Considering their aggressive nature, increased human encounters and worsening envenomation events are likely.[19]

Counter to the Africanized honeybee, the domestic European honeybee is experiencing a withdrawal of range. *Apis mellifera* is a species that has demonstrated great adaptability to many climactic environments in that it can be found almost everywhere in the world.[21] A *mellifera* is instrumental as insect pollinators. Approximately 35% of agricultural crops and 84% of cultivated plant species are reliant on honeybees for pollination.[21] Since 1995, mortality of honeybees worldwide has been observed. The consensus is that this is related to a combination of factors. In addition to pesticides, which kill many colonies each year, there are factors linked to climate change leading to environmental stress, as well as new pathogens such as the brood parasite, *Varroa destructor*. Other factors, such as mismatches between phenology of honeybee colonies and flowering plants, have also had a significant impact on colony health and increased bee mortality.[21–25] It is thought that these factors that might interfere with the honeybees' capability to adapt to climate warming.[25,26]

The mason bee, genus *Osmia* sp, order Hymenoptera, pose little to no threat of stinging because males do not have a stinger, and the females will only sting if threatened. Though not a significant direct health risk, such as anaphylaxis, they are very

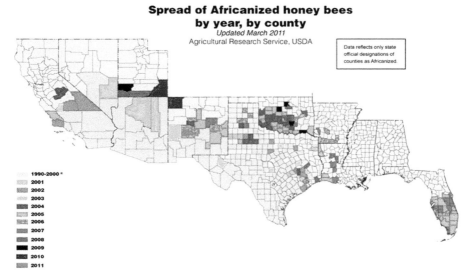

Fig. 1. Spread of Africanized honeybees. (*From* Agricultural Research Service. Spread of Africanized honey bees by year, by county. US Department of Agriculture. Available at: https://www.ars.usda.gov/ARSUserFiles/20220500/New%20Bee%20Map09%20compressed. jpg Accessed March 23, 2020; with permission.)

important pollinators. Using 17 climate chambers, Frund and colleagues[27] demonstrated that overwintering temperature did not influence mortality, which was uniformly low. They did demonstrate that overwintering temperature affected both weight loss after winter and the date of emergence. Weight loss reflects higher metabolic rates during overwintering at warmer temperatures and ultimately resulting in loss of energy, consequently increasing vulnerability and decreasing longevity of wild bees. These findings may further explain reduction of bee populations.

BUMBLEBEES (*BOMBUS* SP.)

There are more than 250 species within the genus *Bombus*, part of the family Apidae. Bumble bees are found in both the Northern and Southern Hemisphere, predominantly in cooler alpine climates.[28] Bumblebees are uncommon causes of sting reactions but have been reported to cause anaphylaxis, particularly with occupational exposure in greenhouse workers.[8,29] Bumblebees have been in decline since the early 1900s. Early loss was initially attributed to loss of habitat for feeding and nesting resources.[28] Marshall and colleagues[30] studied 48 *Bombus* species common to Europe, using applied modeling with climate change scenarios. Analysis projected that by 2100 most of the bumblebee species will lose range, whereas some may experience a slight gain of range. A Belgium study[31] looked at heat stress tolerance of bumblebees, 2 taxa with an arctic distribution, 3 mountainous taxa, and 1 widespread taxon. Relatively low tolerance to heat stress was seen in all groups, with least tolerance in arctic species. These data suggest that heatwaves could lead to fatal consequences for bumblebee species.[31] In a recent study published in *Science*, Soroye and colleagues[32] studied 66 species of bumblebees in North America and Europe, estimating the thermal and precipitation limits of each of the species. The data provided evidence of rapid and widespread declines of bumblebees across Europe and North America, with decreases of 46% in North America and 17% in Europe. They concluded that climate change has driven stronger and more widespread bumblebee declines than previously reported.[32] Unlike many other taxa, bumblebees have failed to track warming, resulting in losses in their southern range and failure to expand in northern range in both Europe and North America, accumulating range compression in both continents.[33] Therefore, bumblebees are vulnerable to further and possible accelerated decline due to climate change, adding further concern to cultivated plant pollination.

Although not a high risk with regard to anaphylaxis, it is important to note that some Hymenoptera species, particularly bees, may not be able to expand range or adapt to the changing climate. Although this will likely decrease human encounters, it could have a significant impact on pollination.

ANTS (FORMICIDAE)

The family Formicidae is composed of more than 14,000 species. Within the genus *Solenopsis*, 2 species, *Solenopsis invicta* and *Solenopsi richteri* have become economically and medically important pests in the United States, with *S invicta* responsible for 95% of sting reactions from ants in North America. Commonly referred to as imported fire ants or invasive fire ants (IFA), they build very large sub-terrarium nests with large mounds. Highly aggressive, they can sting multiple times in a circular pattern, producing sterile pseudo-pustules, and in some, potentially severe, life-threatening anaphylaxis.[8] There are other species of stinging ants throughout most continents. In the United States, the distribution of *S invicta* and *S. richteri* is predominantly in the Southeastern region (**Fig. 2**).

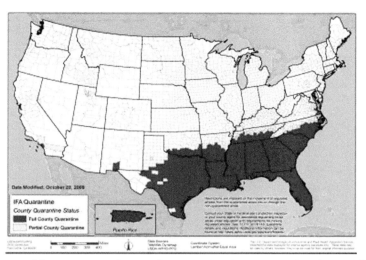

Fig. 2. Imported fire ant quarantine, as of June 9, 2017. (*From* Agricultural Research Service. Imported Fire Ant Quarantine. US Department of Agriculture. Available at: https://www. aphis.usda.gov/aphis/ourfocus/planthealth/plant-pest-and-disease-programs/pests-and-diseases/imported-fire-ants/ct_imported_fire_ants Accessed March 23, 2020; with permission.)

IFAs are invasive species in the United States. Native to South America, *S invicta* was accidently introduced to the Southern United States in the 1930s and again in 1945 and has successfully increased its range to include the Southeastern Region and Southern California, as depicted in **Fig. 2**.[34,35] *S richteri* was introduced into the United States in the 1950s, although with a much small footprint.

Using scientific modeling, it is predicted that changing climate will create favorable conditions for further northern expansion. Morrison and colleagues[35] predicted northern range expansion of *S invicta* of 80 to 150 km, with acceleration of expansion by the second half of the twenty-first century. This was modeled using Vegetation-Ecosystem Modeling and Analysis Project (VEMAP) along with historical data from the North American Oceanic and Atmospheric Administration. VEMAP is a multi-institutional, international effort whose goal is to evaluate the sensitivity of terrestrial ecosystem and vegetation processes to altered climate forcing and elevated atmospheric CO_2 (Vegetation-Ecosystem Modeling and Analysis Project [VEMAP] Available at: DAAC Home > Get Data > NASA Projects > Vegetation-Ecosystem Modeling and Analysis Project [VEMAP]. Accessed March 18, 2020) Findings revealed that in some areas, expansion range of IFA would be limited by drier conditions, while range increased in higher elevations where temperatures are cooler.[35]

It is projected that *S invicta* will continue to expand its range within the United States, at least in part due to climate warming. This will undoubtably increase insect-human contact. Based on a prospective study, sting rate with exposure is more than 50% and the potential development of allergic sensitivity is 7%.[36] Thus, in addition to economic impact, the continued spread of imported fire ants will almost certainly result in increased morbidity and mortality risk.

Pachycondyla chinensis, or the Asian needle ant, is native to areas of Japan and Asia. Like the imported fire ant, it is in the order Hymenoptera and family Formicidae. The Asian needle ant is another invasive species in the United States. It was first introduced in North Carolina early in the twentieth century and is rapidly spreading along the Eastern United States and throughout a wide range of habitats.[37,38] Stings from the Asian needle ant are an important cause of anaphylaxis in East Asia. A 23-kDa protein homologous to antigen 5 is the major allergen produced by these ants.[39] Using species distribution models, Bertelsmeier and colleagues,[38] demonstrated that climate change will greatly increase the risk of *P chinenis* invasion by increasing suitable landmass by 64.9% worldwide. Climate change is a crucial factor in extending the habitat of this invasive ant. There is concern over anaphylaxis risk to this stinging insect that we lack the ability to perform venom testing and are unable to offer immunotherapy.

LEPIDOPTERA
Caterpillars/Butterflies/Moths

Lepidoptera are "scaly, winged insects," comprising butterflies and moths in all stages of development. There are an estimated 140,000 species in this class. They have a very complex life cycle: however, a general understanding is important. After the male and female mate, the fertilized eggs are deposited onto foliage, where they hatch, and the larval form (caterpillar) emerges. The caterpillar undergoes 5 or 6 developmental molts and transformations known as instars. It is during these early developmental stages that they are a threat to humans. The most mature instar pupates into a cocoon, ultimately emerging as an adult.[40,41] Lepidopterism and erucism are interchangeable terms that refers to the ill effects of larval and adult butterflies and moths resulting from inhalation, ingestion, direct contact, or envenomation. The stinging or urticating caterpillars excrete their venom through hollow hairs or spines, which can result in hypersensitivity reactions, including local and/or systemic reactions. Caterpillars excrete their venom through hollow hairs or spines. As an example, during the final instar of *Euproctis similis*, there are an estimated 2,000,000 urticating setae per caterpillar.[40,42,43]

There are an estimated 50 to 150 species that have been implicated in lepidopterism, representing only 0.1% of the known species of moths and butterflies. Four species of caterpillar frequently encountered in the United States pose a potentially serious threat for the sensitized victim: (1) the io moth caterpillar (*Automeris io*); (2) the saddleback caterpillar (*Sibine stimulea*); (3) the Douglas fir tussock moth caterpillar (*Orgyia pseudotsugata*); and (4) the puss caterpillar or "asp" (*Megalopyge opercularis*). These have all been reported as causing serious occupational and public health problems, related to lepidioterism.[40,41] Because of their quick response to climactic factors, butterflies are good indicators of climate change in Europe. The Butterfly Monitoring Scheme has accurate data sets dating back to the 1970s. As of 2005, the average temperature in Europe had increased 0.8° C. With that change, 63% of butterfly species expanded their range northward.[44,45]

Expansion of range of Lepidoptera in response to climate change provides information that is helpful in assessing redistribution of other insects, which in turn is an important demonstration of potential impacts on human health. This is demonstrated in a meta-analysis, Battisti and colleagues[46] reported that over the past 20 years there has been an increase in reporting of setae-related health problems associated with expansion of the processionary moth. The processionary moth, subfamily Thaumetopoea, consists of approximately 100 species, occurring across Africa, Asia, Europe, Australia, and the Middle East.[46]

SUMMARY

Frazier and colleagues[47] reported on the relationship between increasing temperatures and population growth of 65 insect species. Insects that adapt well to warmer environments experienced an increase in population growth rates. Deutsch and colleagues[48] in turn demonstrated that with a warming climate, the fitness of ectothermic organisms is expected to generally increase with their latitude. Based on these data, faster population growth for insects at mid to high latitudes, and negative consequences with increased extinction rates for ectothermic species near the equator has been forecast.

Anticipating how climate change will affect cyclic and seasonal patterns across latitudes as temperatures increase will be determined by the thermal sensitivities and tolerance of insect species. Expansion of range toward the poles has been demonstrated in many species. As discussed in this review, most insects known to cause anaphylaxis are predicted to expand their range, thereby almost certainly increasing the frequency of human encounters.

Some species may be less adaptable or less tolerant and move toward extinction. This has been demonstrated in both honeybees and bumblebees.[21–25,32,33] As discussed, the expansion of range for social wasps has been documented through modeling, predicting a continuation of this trend of expansion of range. There are other studies that suggest there could be a decrease in social wasp expansion, in part due to reduced ability to defend against parasitoids, bacteria, and viruses, and to intolerance of greater rainfall as a result of climactic changes.[49]

Although beyond the scope of this review, synchrony between the insect and its environment is of great importance. Insects are key to pollination of many plants, with almost 88% of angiosperms relying on insects for pollination services (entomophilous). Much work has been focused on shifts in flowering time and insect emergence and potential temporal mismatches between the two.[25,26]

It is likely that climate change will continue to alter the distribution and population of Hymenoptera and other insects. As temperatures warm and regions become suitable for nesting and establishment of colonies, many insects will expand their territory. It is the job of the allergist/immunologist to recognize these changing patterns and to educate and manage the human impact of our changing climate.

DISCLOSURE

The author has nothing to disclose.

REFERENCES

1. Boggs C. The fingerprints of global climate change on insect populations. Curr Opin Sci 2016;17:69–73.
2. Wuebbles DJ, Fahey DW, Hubbard KA, et al. 2017: Executive summary. In: Wuebbles DJ, Fahey DW, Hubbard KA, et al, editors. Climate science special report: fourth national climate assessment, Vol I. Washington, DC: U.S. Global Change Research Program; 2017. p. 12–34. https://doi.org/10.7930/J0DJ5RG.
3. Beggs PJ. Introduction. In: Beggs PJ, editor. Impacts of climate change on allergens and allergic disease. Cambridge (United Kingdom): Cambridge University Press; 2016. p. 1–9.
4. Haahtela T. The biodiversity hypothesis. Allergy 2019;74(8):1445–56.
5. Haahtela T, Akdis C, Benjaponpitak S, et al. The biodiversity hypothesis and allergic disease: a statement: paper of the World Allergy Organization. World Allergy Organ J 2013;6(3). https://doi.org/10.1186/1939-4551-6-3.
6. Davis A, Jenkinson LS, Laton JH, et al. Making mistakes when predicting shifts in species range in response to global warming. Nature 1998;391:783–6.

7. Needleman RK, Neylan IP, Erickson T. Potential environmental and ecological effects of global climate change on venomous terrestrial species in the wilderness. Wilderness Environ Med 2018;29(2):226–38.

8. Golden DBK, Demain JG, Freeman T, et al. Stinging insect hypersensitivity: a proactivity: a practice parameter update 2016. Ann Allergy Asthma Immunol 2017; 118(1):28–54.

9. Lester PJ, Beggs JR. Invasion success and management strategies for social *Vespula* wasps. Annu Rev Entomol 2019;64:51–71.

10. Turillazzi S, Turillazzi F. Climate changes and Hymenoptera venom allergy: are there some connections? Curr Opin Allergy Clin Immunol 2017;17(5):344–9.

11. Oswalt ML, Foote JT, Kemp SF. Anaphylaxis: Report of two fatal yellowjacket stings in Alaska. J Allergy Clin Immunol 2007;119(1):534.

12. Demain JG, Gessner BD. Increasing incidence of medical visits due to insect sting in Alaska. Alaska Epidemiology Bulletin 2008;13.

13. Demain JG, Gessner B, McLaughlin J, et al. Increasing insect reactions in Alaska: is this related to climate change? Allergy Asthma Proc 2009;30:238–43.

14. CBC News. Rare sightings of wasp north of Arctic Circle puzzles residents. 2004. Available at: http://www.cbc.ca/health/story/2004/09/09/wasp040909.html. Accessed March 17, 2020.

15. Barnes BM, Barger JL, Seares J, et al. Overwintering in yellowjacket queens (*Vespula vulgaris*) and green stinkbugs (*Elasmostethus interstincus*) in subarctic Alaska. Physiol Zool 1996;69:1469–80.

16. Lester PJ, Haywood J, Archer ME, et al. The long-term population dynamics of the common wasps in their native and invading range. J Anim Ecol 2017;86: 337–47.

17. Hocherl N, Tautz J. Nesting behavior of the paper wasp Pollistes in Central Europe-a flexible system for expanding into new areas. Ecosphere 2015;6:1–11.

18. Barbet-Mason M, Rome Q, Muller F, et al. Climate change increases the risk of invasion by the Yellow-legged hornet. J Bio Con 2013;157:4–10.

19. Vega A, Castro L. Impact of climate change on insect-human interactions. Curr Opin Allergy Clin Immunol 2019;19(5):475–81.

20. Schumacher MJ, Schmidt JO, Egen NB, et al. Biochemical variability of venoms from individual European and Africanized honeybees. J Allergy Clin Immunol 1992;90(1):59–65.

21. Conte YL, Navajas M. Climate change: impact on honeybee populations and diseases. Rev Sci Tech 2008;27(2):485–97, 499-510.

22. Oldroyd BP. What's killing American honeybees. PLoS Biol 2007;5(6):168.

23. Pettis J, Vanengelsdrop D, Cox-Foster D. Colony collapse disorder working group pathogen sub-group report. Am Bee J 2007;147(7):595–7.

24. Vanengelsdrop D, Evans JD, Saegerman C, et al. Colony collapse disorder: A descriptive study. PLoS One 2009;4(8):e6481.

25. Nurnberger F, Hartel S, Steffan-Dewenter I. Seasonal timing in honeybee colonies: phenology shifts affect honey stores and varroa infestation levels. Oecologia 2019;189(4):1121–31.

26. Ollerton J, Winfree R, Tarrant S. How many flowering plants are pollinated by animals? Oikos 2011;120:321–6.

27. Frund J, Zieger SL, Tscharntke T. Response diversity of wild bees to overwintering temperature. Oecologia 2013;173:1639–48.

28. Condamine FL, Hines HM. Historical species losses in bumblebee evolution. Biol Lett 2015;11(3):20141049.

29. deGroot H. Allergy to bumblebees. Curr Opin Allergy Clin Immunol 2006;6:294–7.

30. Marshall L, Biesmeijer JC, Rasmont P, et al. The interplay of climate and land use change affects the distribution of EU bumblebees. Glob Chang Biol 2018;24(1): 101–16.
31. Martinet B, Lecocq T, Smet J, et al. A protocol to assess insect resistance to heat waves, applied to bumblebees (Bombus Latreille, 1802). PLoS One 2015;10(3): e0118591.
32. Soroye P, Newbol T, Kerr J. Climate change contributes to widespread declines among bumble bees across continents. Science 2020;367(6478):685–8.
33. Kerr JT, Pindar A, Galpern P, et al. Climate change impacts on bumblebees converge across continents. Science 2015;349(6244):177–80.
34. Morrison LW, Porter SD, Daniels E, et al. Potential global range expansion of the invasive fire ant, *Solenopsis invicta*. Biol Invasions 2004;6:183–91.
35. Morrison LW, Korzukhin MD, Porter SD. Predicted range expansion on invasive fire ant, Solenopsis invictis, in eastern United States based on the VEMAP global warming scenario. Diversity Distrib 2005; 11:199-204.
36. Tracy JM, Demain JG, Quinn JM, et al. The natural history of imported fire ant (*Solenopsis invicta*). J Allergy Clin Immunol 1995;95(4):824–8.
37. Guenard BB, Dunn RR. A new (old) invasive ant in the hardwood forests of Eastern North Carolina and its potentially widespread impacts. PLoS One 2010;5(7):e11614.
38. Bertelsmeier C, Guenard B, Courchamp F. Climate change may boost the invasion of the Asian needle ant. PLoS One 2013;8(10):e75438.
39. Jeong KY, Yi MH, Son M, et al. IgE Reactivity of Recombinant Pac c 3 from the Asian Needle Ant (Pachycondyla chinensis). Int Arch Allergy Immunol 2016; 169:93–100.
40. Wirtz RA. Allergic and toxic reaction to non-stinging arthropods. Annu Rev Entomol 1984;29:47–69.
41. Rosen T. Caterpillar dermatitis. Dermatol Clin 1990;8:245–52.
42. Beck EC. Identification of insects that affect human health. Cutis 1977;19:781–4.
43. Biery TL. Venomous arthropod handbook. Washington, DC: US Government Printing Office; 1978. p. 1–36.
44. Vickey M. Butterflies as indicators of climate change. Sci Prog 2008;91(2): 193–201.
45. Dell D, Sparks TH, Dennis RLH. Climate change and the effect of increasing spring temperatures on emergence dates of the butterfly Apatura iris (Lepidoptera: Nymphalidae). Eur J Entomol 2005;102(2):161–7.
46. Battisti A, Larsson S, Roques A. Processionary moths and associated urtication risk: global change-driven effects. Annu Rev Entomol 2017;62:323–42.
47. Frazier M, Huey R, Berrigan D. Thermodynamics constrains the insect population growth rates: "warmer is better. Am Nat 2006;168(4):512–20.
48. Deutsch CA, Tewksbury JJ, Huey RB, et al. Impacts of climate warming on terrestrial ectotherms across latitude. Proc Natl Acad Sci U S A 2008;105(18):6668–72.
49. Dejean A, Cereghino R, Carpenter JM, et al. Climate change impact on neotropical social wasps. PLoS One 2011;6(11):e27004.

The Impact of Climate Change on Pollen Season and Allergic Sensitization to Pollens

Young-Jin Choi, MD, PhD[a], Kyung Suk Lee, MD, PhD[a,b], Jae-Won Oh, MD, PhD[a,b],*

KEYWORDS

• Climate change • Allergy • Sensitization • Pollen • Pollination

KEY POINTS

• Climate change may affect the seasonal allergic diseases due to longer pollen seasons and increase both allergic sensitization and symptom prevalence with severity.
• The complex interaction of air pollution and temperature on pollen production and allergenicity makes the overall risk assessment of tree pollens challenging.
• The future direction of research on climate change is speculative, because the influence on humans is complex.

INTRODUCTION

Climate change represents a massive threat to global health that could affect many disease factors in the twenty-first century. Among previous reports, climate change influences the development of asthma and allergic diseases and influences pollen productions that induce allergic manifestations.[1-4] The influence of a changing climate on allergic disease has generated interest from the public and the scientific community. The climate is constantly changing and variable over time and is dependent on incoming solar radiation, outgoing thermal radiation, and the composition of the atmosphere on earth. Climate change is a constant process that affects allergy. Impacts on pollen may be one of the most important consequences of climate change for human health.[1] There are multiple interrelated, potential consequences of climatic change on plant phenology. Therefore, the change subsequently can influence the occurrence of

[a] Department of Pediatrics, Hanyang University Guri Hospital, 153 Gyungchun-Ro, Guri, Gyunggi-Do 11923, South Korea; [b] Department of Pediatrics, College of Medicine, Hanyang University, Seoul, South Korea
* Corresponding author. Department of Pediatrics, Hanyang University Guri Hospital, 153 Gyungchun-Ro, Guri, Gyunggi-Do 11923, South Korea.
E-mail address: jaewonoh@hanyang.ac.kr

Immunol Allergy Clin N Am 41 (2021) 97–109
https://doi.org/10.1016/j.iac.2020.09.004   immunology.theclinics.com
0889-8561/21/© 2020 Elsevier Inc. All rights reserved.

pollen allergy. Especially respiratory allergic disease, such as asthma, allergic rhinitis (AR), allergic conjunctivitis (AC), and even atopic dermatitis, will increase under climate change in part because of the impact on allergenic plant species.[2,3] Pollens are a major cause of symptoms in allergic individuals, but because the influence of climate change is complex, there is no predictable quantitative assessment of how climate change may affect the levels of pollen allergy in humans in the future.[4] For example, an altered climate will affect the range of allergenic plant species as well as the length of the pollen season, and elevated atmospheric carbon dioxide (CO_2) may increase plant productivity and pollen production.[5] Climate change also may affect the release and atmospheric dispersion of pollen.[2] The overall impact will be alteration of pollen season timing and load and, hence, changes in exposure. Modeling all of these processes is needed to evaluate the consequences of climate change on pollen-related allergic disease.

The future consequences of these trends are speculative, but the allergy community must be knowledgeable about the issues; understand the anticipatable effect on allergic diseases, including asthma, AR, and AC; and be well-versed in possible means to mitigate adverse health consequences. The public and scientific community has generally interested in The influence of future climate on pollen allergy.[5,6] Most studies on the impact of climate change on aeroallergens can be divided into pollen amount, pollen allergenicity, pollen season, distribution of allergic plants, and pollen.[7,8] Several research articles on climate change effects on distributions of allergenic pollens have focused typically on analysis of observed pollen counts and their regression relationships with local meteorologic factors.[9–11] There are 3 major issues by which climate change could influence allergic disease. First, warmer temperatures and a longer pollen season could increase the duration of human exposure to aeroallergens with consequences for increased allergic sensitization.[12] The dates of phenological events, such as the release of pollen and subsequent bud burst, could be the same after climatic warming. In warmer weather, bud bursting would occur slightly earlier but would require a greater thermal time in order for the risk of frost damage to be the same. Second, climate change could increase the level of allergenic airborne pollen and allergic symptoms associated with exposure. The onset, duration of pollination, and abundance of pollen grains in the air vary from year to year. Finally, climate disruptions with air pollution and/or increased CO_2 and the other greenhouse gases might change allergen concentration of the pollen and alter the allergenicity and its symptom severity.[13,14] Weather variables, mainly air temperature, sunlight, and rainfall, together with CO_2 are among the main factors affecting phenology, which means the times of the appearance of first leaves, first flowers, autumn leaf coloration, and so on and pollen production by plant. In addition, weather patterns influence the movement and dispersion of all aeroallergens in the atmosphere through the action of winds and rainfall and depend on the atmospheric stability.[15,16] The relationships between changing start dates for pollen seasons, which immediately precede bud burst, and changing spring temperatures provide an indication of the current status of the response to future changes in spring temperatures, although the start of the pollen season may be influenced by factors affecting pollen dispersal, such as rainfall or lack of wind.[10,17,18] Monitoring pollen must be recorded with meteorologic variables when pollen is in the air and when pollen matures on the plants for the evaluation of pollination.

WEATHER AND POLLEN SEASON

Plants basically require a certain amount of heat to complete their development; then, air temperature plays a key role, together with day length, water and nutrient availability, soil type, and so forth. Therefore, weather conditions, including rainfall, humidity, wind speed, and air temperature, may alter the concentrations of pollens. Increasing worldwide evidence demonstrates that the timing of life-cycle events of a large number of plants have responded to the increase in air temperature. Increased temperatures may lead to earlier pollination of many plants and longer duration of pollination. Several species have been shown to produce more pollen with warmer temperatures. Additionally, climate change is thought to increase the quantity of allergenic protein that individual pollen grains contain. Changes also involve plants producing allergenic pollen, with expected consequences on allergic individuals.[19–23] Longer pollen seasons increase duration of exposure, potentially resulting in more sensitization. Longer pollen seasons also lead to longer symptomatic periods in those with allergic disease, and higher pollen concentrations may lead to more severe symptoms. An earlier start of pollen season was confirmed in studies focused on allergenic plant. Due to the earlier onset, the pollen seasons are interrupted more often by adverse weather conditions in late winter or early spring.[13,17,24–30] Duration of the pollen season also is extended, especially in summer and in late flowering species. Moreover, there is some evidence of significantly stronger allergenicity in pollen from trees growing at increased temperatures.[28,29]

Several studies regarding the relationship between climate change and pollen allergy have indicated that plant phenology is shifting in response to global warming.[30–32] Research about trends in pollen concentrations, however, has focused either on limited site-specific studies or on a single source or small subset of allergenic pollen taxa, such as ragweed, across a larger geographic area, with several studies varying with respect to temporal increases in pollen season duration or pollen load.[33–35] Hence, along-term analysis of compound allergenic plant species across different continents and different environmental regimes is needed to assess whether recent climate-induced changes are affecting seasonal exposure to airborne pollen on a global scale. Cumulative pollen concentrations and a preset percentage threshold level are used to define the start and end of the pollen season. The start of the pollen season can be defined as the point when the cumulative pollen count reaches 5% of the annual pollen integral, the yearly cumulative count, and the end of the season defined as the point when the count reaches 95%.

Analyses of recent trends that include multiple pollen sources across large geographic areas are scarce. Ziello and colleagues[36] analyzed data set consisting of 1221 pollen time series at 97 locations in 13 European countries from 23 pollen taxa across 97 stations in Europe, but most stations had pollen records ranging from 10 to 28 years. A tendency toward an increase in pollen was noted; however, substantial variability in the seasonal pollen index, and no significant correlation between seasonal trends and mean air temperature was reported. Zhang and colleagues[37] presented a similar spatiotemporal analysis within the United States; they also reported increasing trends in seasonality and pollen amounts for a subset of allergenic plants, such as birch, oak, ragweed, mugwort, and grass, over a 17-year period. Although a significant correlation with latitude was observed, correlations between temperature and pollen seasonality or load were not established. Overall, the long-term data indicate significant increases in both pollen loads and pollen season duration over time across the pollen collection locations, although without a clear latitudinal trend. Recently, analysis from Ziska and colleagues[38] illustrates a clear positive correlation between recent global warming and an increase in the seasonal duration and amount of pollen for multiple allergenic plant species on a decadal basis for the northern hemisphere. If the change in pollen load over time for a given location is compared with the temporal change in either maximum temperature (Tmax) or minimum temperature (Tmin), 12 (71%) of the 17 locations showed significant increases in seasonal cumulative pollen or annual pollen load. Similarly, 11 (65%) of the 17 locations showed a significant increase in pollen season duration over time, increasing, on average, 0.9 days per year. Across the northern hemisphere locations analyzed, annual cumulative increases in Tmax over time were significantly associated with percentage increases in seasonal pollen load as were annual cumulative increases in Tmin. A significant association is observed in the present study, indicating that temperature contributed to seasonal changes in pollen load on a global level (**Fig. 1**). Changes in Tmax and Tmin for cumulative degree day were significant (**Fig. 2**). The lengthening of pollen seasons is related to both earlier springs and later autumns. Although the increase in temperature is known to vary with latitude, its impact on the increase in pollen concentrations, in terms of intensity and duration, appears to be global and independent of latitude.[38] These data indicate that recent climatic changes, through temperature, are affecting pollen amounts as well as season duration and timing in the northern hemisphere.

These observed changes may implicate the future respiratory allergic diseases, such as AR and asthma. Future climate projections also suggest changes in the duration of the pollen season and an estimated rising in sensitization to allergenic plants, such as ragweed.[39,40] Similarly, projections for other allergenic species, such as oak, indicate that a longer duration of the pollen season might be related to increased emergency department visits in future in the United States.[41] Hazards are naturally occurring physical events that can have an impact on human health both directly and indirectly through disarrangement to ecosystems and the services they provide with climate-driven shifts in their distribution, frequency, and intensity. In contrast to the depth of knowledge available for anthropogenic-related threats, climate change drivers can interact in synergistic ways, yet the interactive effect of global change drivers on plant pollination are poorly represented in several previous studies.[41,42] For illuminating global change drivers, a study paired manipulative experiments to probe 2 mechanistic pathways through which plant invasion and global warming may alter phenology and reproduction of native plant species. They tested how experimental warming ($+1.7°C$) modulated flowering phenology and how this affected flowering overlap between a native plant and an invasive plant. The flowering overlap of native and invasive plants would be altered by warming, given that invading plants typically exhibit greater phenological plasticity than native plants. These results illustrate a pathway through which global change drivers can operate synergistically to alter pollination.[41]

SENSITIZATION TO ALLERGIC POLLEN

Hypersensitivity to pollens is one of the most common aspects of the allergic disease, leading to AR, AC, and asthma.[42] Subjects with pollen allergy can be sensitized to a single or to several pollen species, depending on their exposure to regional pollens.[43] Sensitization to multiple allergens, including pollens, has been reported to lead to more serious allergic symptoms and to increase the risk of asthma.[44–46] An interaction between the exposure to pollen and being sensitized to pollen allergens was detected that the effect was less pronounced in individuals who were sensitized to only 1 type of pollen, compared with who are sensitized to all types of pollen (trees, grasses, and weeds).[47] Furthermore, because different pollen types are released at different periods of the pollen season, atopic individuals sensitized to more than o1ne type of pollen are experiencing a longer period of exposure, which may lead to a stronger effect on airway hyperreactivity and reduced lung function.[47]

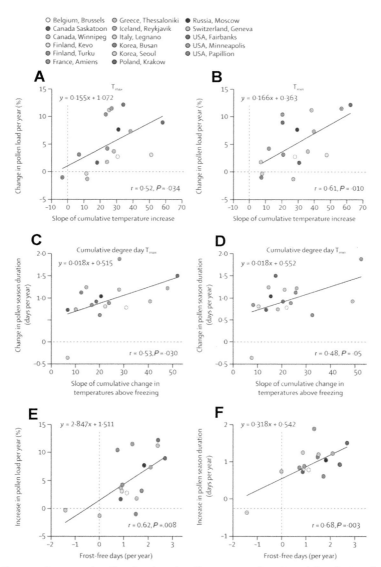

Fig. 1. Changes in annual pollen load and pollen season duration. (*A*) Relative change in annual pollen load as a function of slope of cumulative Tmax by location over time. (*B*) Relative change in annual pollen load as a function of slope of cumulative Tmin by location over time. (*C*) Change in pollen season duration as a function of the cumulative degree day above freezing for Tmax by location over time. (*D*) Change in pollen season duration as a function of the cumulative degree day higher than the freezing point for Tmin by location over time. (*E*) Average annual percentage change in pollen load as a function of temporal changes in frost-free days by location. (*F*) Average annual percentage change in pollen season duration as a function of temporal changes in frost-free days by location. (*From* Ziska LH, Makra PL, Harry SK, et al. Temperature-related changes in airborne allergenic pollen abundance and seasonality across the northern hemisphere: a retrospective data analysis. Lancet Planet Health. 2019;3:e124-131; Reprinted with permission from Elsevier.)

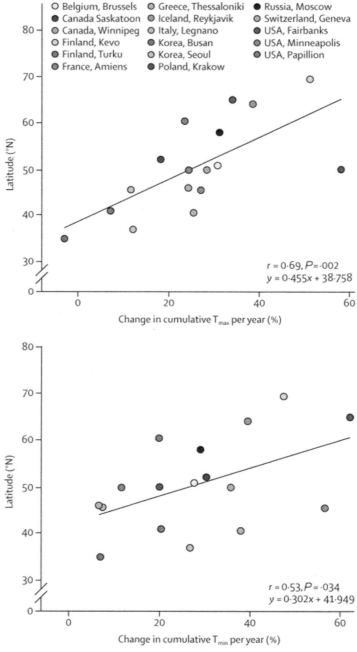

Fig. 2. Change over time in cumulative Tmax (*top panel*) and Tmin (*bottom panel*) for each of the 17 locations used in the study as a function of latitude. (*From* Ziska LH, Makra PL, Harry SK, et al. Temperature-related changes in airborne allergenic pollen abundance and seasonality across the northern hemisphere: a retrospective data analysis. Lancet Planet Health. 2019;3:e124-131; Reprinted with permission from Elsevier.)

There is the different threshold level of allergic sensitization among plant species. Because the threshold level of grass pollen concentration needed to develop allergy symptoms is considered to be significantly lower than the corresponding level for birch, it may be taken more days with pollen levels above this threshold for grass than for birch pollen.[48] In previous studies, an increase in sensitivity to grass pollen has been observed as the pollen season progresses.[49] Subjects who perceived allergen sensitization were more likely to have actual sensitization to at least 1 aeroallergen; 83.9% perceived allergen sensitization to at least 1 outdoor allergen. A US study of 247 adults with asthma found no significant correlation between reported allergic symptoms to pollens and skin prick test (SPT) wheal size to pollens and mild correlation for reported pet allergy and SPT wheal size to cat and dog.[50] In contrast, a separate Finnish study of 290 young adults found that reported AR from pollen or animal dander and furs had a specificity and sensitivity of 87% for sensitization to any allergen by serum IgE or SPT.[51]

There are multiple interrelated, potential consequences of climatic change on respiratory allergic disease. Rising air temperatures can influence pollen season duration with commensurate changes in the duration of human exposure to aeroallergens and plant distribution with allergenic mixtures. Warmer temperature might increase seasonal intensity of the allergenic load and the concentration of pollen. These changes are important, given that the duration of the pollen season is correlated with the duration of symptomatic periods among atopic individuals and that allergenic pollen concentration is positively correlated with symptom severity at a population level. Climate change could alter the allergenicity or allergen concentration of the pollen.[19,52] Overall, climate changes in contact to allergenic pollens are likely to affect both sensitization rates and allergic symptom prevalence and severity.[2,3,53]

POLLUTION AND POLLINATION

Environmental and meteorologic changes, driven by increased concentrations of greenhouse gases, have widespread impacts on biotic systems, including direct and indirect effects on human health.[54] Several studies have suggested that traffic-related pollutants can disrupt pollen, a modification that aggravate allergic symptoms.[13,55–57] In particular, it has been suggested that particulate matter (PM) may interact with aeroallergens, promoting airway sensitization by modulating the allergenicity of pollen.[58] Several epidemiologic studies have investigated the synergic effects of air pollution and pollen exposure on rhinitis symptoms, with conflicting findings.[59,60] Different models suggest that an increase in the concentration of atmospheric CO_2 is one of the most certain predictors of climate change. The CO_2 concentration has increased by 29% since preindustrial times. The average tropospheric CO_2 concentration has risen from 290 parts per million (ppm) in 1850 (preindustrial era) to 353 ppm in 1990.[61] Over the past 50 years, the global earth temperature has risen markedly. Approximately 75% of the anthropogenic CO_2 emissions to the atmosphere during the past 50 years resulted from fossil fuel burning.[62] The key determinants of greenhouse gas emissions are energy production, transportation, agriculture, food production, and waste management. Moreover, rising temperatures contribute to the elevation of the concentrations of ozone (O_3) and PM with CO_2 at ground level.[63,64] Urbanization and high levels of vehicle emission have been shown to increase the frequency of seasonal respiratory allergy in people living in urban areas in comparison with those living in rural areas.[65] Published data suggest an increasing effect of aeroallergens on allergic patients, leading to a greater likelihood of development of an allergic respiratory disease in sensitized patients and an aggravation in patients already symptomatic.[27,66]

Increasing CO_2 and temperature seem to substantially increase pollen production from ragweed in experimental conditions. The same results were obtained in a study on ragweed plants growing in urban and rural areas, providing a natural model for evaluating possible effects of global warming. Some studies showed that Amb a 1 concentration in ragweed pollen increased as a function of CO_2 concentration. The difference in Amb a 1 as a result of increased CO_2 also may be affected by influences among and within different ragweed populations.[10,67,68] Furthermore, ragweed pollen collected along high-traffic roads showed a higher allergen city due to traffic-related pollution. Pollen from birch trees exposed to higher O_3 levels induces larger wheals and flares in SPT compared with lower O_3-exposed pollen, suggesting an allergenicity increasing effect of O_3.[27,68] Other factors, however, might modify the distribution of allergenic plants in Europe. The cases of grass and ragweed are explanatory. Grass pollen is responsible for a high portion of pollen allergy worldwide, and variations in total pollen count have been observed in past decades. Rogers and colleagues[25] reported faster growth of spikes as a result of high CO_2 concentrations over a limited period of time. Furthermore, Kim and colleagues[69] recently presented the oak trees under the elevated CO_2 levels, which are expected in the changing climate, produced significantly higher amount of pollen and allergenic protein than under the present air conditions. The number and weight of oak pollen grains from the CO_2-enriched open-top chamber per plant and per catkin increased from the ambient CO_2 (**Fig. 3, Table 1**). Although there are few reports on the response of tree pollens to CO_2 concentrations, these results are supported by those of other studies on weed species.[69] The analysis of the time series of aerobiological data from the United Kingdom, the longest of the world, showed a decreasing trend in terms of yearly grass pollen counts and severity of pollen season and an earlier start of the season. There are remarkable differences between the 3 study sites, however, underlining the role of local determinants, such as meteorologic factors, plant adaptation, changes in land use, and changes in species

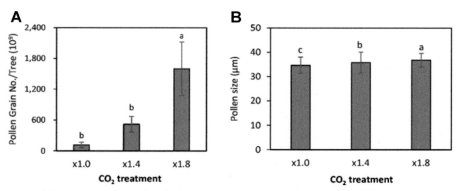

Fig. 3. (*A*) Total number of pollen grains and (*B*) mean diameter of the pollen grains collected from the CO_2 open-top chambers, ×1.0 CO_2, ×1.4 CO_2, and ×1.8 CO_2 concentrations; ×1.0 CO_2, ×1.4 CO_2, and ×1.8 CO_2 expresses 400 ppm, 560 ppm, and 720 ppm of CO_2 concentrations, respectively. Different lowercase letters on the bars indicate significant differences among treatments in OTCs at 5% significance level by Tukey test. Data represent mean ±SD. (*From* Kim KR, Oh JW, Woo SY, et al. Does the increase in ambient CO 2 concentration elevate allergy risks posed by oak pollen? Int J Biometeorol. 2018 Sep;62(9):1587-1594; with permission.)

Table 1
Number of pollen grains per catkin, weight of pollen per catkin, number of pollen grains per tree, pollen size, and allergenic protein content and their ratio to the ×1.0 treatment

Treatment	Grains/ Catkin (10^6)	Ratio	Weight/ Catkin (mg)	Ratio	Grains/Tree (10^9)	Ratio	Size (μm)	Ratio	Allergen Content (ng/mL)	Ratio
×1.0	324.2	1.00	3.50	1.00	114.4	1.00	34.7	1.00	419.7	1.00
×1.4	388.8	1.20	7.05	2.01	518.3	4.53	35.8	1.03	472.2	1.12
×1.8	590.2	1.82	8.91	2.54	1600.7	13.99	36.9	1.06	467.2	1.11
P value	.045		.003		<.001		<.001		.011	

The *P* values from the 1-way ANOVA also are indicated.

and effects of air pollutants.[70] These studies suggested that the complex interaction of CO_2 concentration and temperature on pollen production and allergenicity makes the overall risk assessment of tree pollens a good challenge. Climate change may induce changes in the ecological suitability of allergenic plants, which may result in new allergy symptoms in groups with no previous problems.[4]

Change of weather pattern may increase episodes of long-distance transport of pollutants as well as of pollen grains, such as ragweed, making large-scale circulation patterns as important as regional ones.[71] Over the past decades, many studies have shown changes in the production, dispersion, and allergen content of pollen and that nature of the changes may vary in different regions and species. Climate change is also having an impact on the biogeographical distribution of plants with consequences for the composition of pollen diversity as well as the magnitude and duration of pollen seasons.[5,72]

CLINICAL CARE POINTS

- Climate change may influence pollen season duration, with human exposure to pollen allergens, and increase seasonal intensity of the allergenic load. Sensitization to pollens lead to serious allergic symptoms and to increase the risk of asthma.[44–46]

- Pollen from birch trees exposed to high O_3 levels induces larger wheals and flares in SPTs, suggesting an allergenicity increasing effect of O_3.[27,68] The interaction of CO_2 concentration and temperature on pollen production and allergenicity might imply to aggravate the risk of tree pollens.[67,69]

- Because the influence of climate change is complex, there is no predictable quantitative assessment that climate change may affect the levels of pollen allergy in humans in the future.[4]

Data from Refs.[4,27,44–46,68]

DISCLOSURE

No commercial or financial conflicts of interest for all authors.

REFERENCES

1. Beggs PJ. Adaptation to impacts of climate change on aeroallergens and allergic respiratory diseases. Int J Environ Res Public Health 2010;7(8):3006–21.

2. Bielory L, Lyons K, Goldberg R. Climate change and allergic disease. Curr Allergy Asthma Rep 2012;12(6):485–94.

3. Shea KM, Truckner RT, Weber RW, et al. Climate change and allergic disease. J Allergy Clin Immunol 2008;122(3):443–53 [quiz: 454–5].

4. Reid CE, Gamble JL. Aeroallergens, allergic disease, and climate change: impacts and adaptation. Ecohealth 2009;6(3):458–70.

5. Ziska LH, Beggs PJ. Anthropogenic climate change and allergen exposure: The role of plant biology. J Allergy Clin Immunol 2012;129(1):27–32.

6. Lake IR, Jones NR, Agnew M, et al. Climate change and future pollen allergy in Europe. Environ Health Perspect 2017;125(3):385–91.

7. Beggs PJ. Climate change and biometeorology, the International Society of Biometeorology and its journal: a perspective on the past and a framework for the future. Int J Biometeorol 2014;58(1):1–6.

8. Fitter AH, Fitter RSR. Rapid changes in flowering Time in British Plants. Science 2002;296:1689–91.

9. Cleland EE, Chuine I, Menzel A, et al. Shifting plant phenology in response to global change. Trends Ecol Evol 2007;22(7):357–65.

10. Frei T, Gassner E. Climate change and its impact on birch pollen quantities and the start of the pollen season an example from Switzerland for the period 1969-2006. Int J Biometeorol 2008;52(7):667–74.

11. Sikoparija B, Skjoth CA, Celenk S, et al. Spatial and temporal variations in airborne Ambrosia pollen in Europe. Aerobiologia (Bologna) 2017;33(2):181–9.

12. Ariano R, Canonica GW, Passalacqua G. Possible role of climate changes in variations in pollen seasons and allergic sensitizations during 27 years. Ann Allergy Asthma Immunol 2010;104(3):215–22.

13. Ziska LH, Gebhard DE, Frenz DA, et al. Cities as harbingers of climate change: common ragweed, urbanization, and public health. J Allergy Clin Immunol 2003; 111(2):290–5.

14. El Kelish A, Zhao F, Heller W, et al. Ragweed (Ambrosia artemisiifolia) pollen allergenicity: SuperSAGE transcriptomic analysis upon elevated CO_2 and drought stress. BMC Plant Biol 2014;14(1):176.

15. Garcia-Mozo H, Galan C, Jato V, et al. Quercus pollen season dynamics in the Iberian peninsula: response to meteorological parameters and possible consequences of climate change. Ann Agric Environ Med 2006;13(2):209–24.

16. Emberlin J, Mullins J, Corden J, et al. Regional variations in grass pollen seasons in the UK, long-term trends and forecast models. Clin Exp Allergy 1999;29(3): 347–56.

17. Emberlin J, Detandt M, Gehrig R, et al. Responses in the start of Betula (birch) pollen seasons to recent changes in spring temperatures across Europe. Int J Biometeorol 2002;46(4):159–70.

18. Gioulekas D, Papakosta D, Damialis A, et al. Allergenic pollen records (15 years) and sensitization in patients with respiratory allergy in Thessaloniki, Greece. Allergy 2004;59(2):174–84.

19. D'Amato G, Cecchi L, Bonini S, et al. Allergenic pollen and pollen allergy in Europe. Allergy 2007;62(9):976–90.

20. Smith M, Cecchi L, Skjoth CA, et al. Common ragweed: a threat to environmental health in Europe. Environ Int 2013;61:115–26.

21. Frenguelli G, Passalacqua G, Bonini S, et al. Bridging allergologic and botanical knowledge in seasonal allergy: a role for phenology. Ann Allergy Asthma Immunol 2010;105(3):223–7.

22. Teranishi H, Katoh T, Kenda K, et al. Global warming and the earlier start of the Japanese-cedar (Cryptomeria japonica) pollen season in Toyama, Japan. Aerobiologia 2006;22:90–4.

23. Beggs PJ. Impacts of climate change on aeroallergens: past and future. Clin Exp Allergy 2004;34(10):1507–13.

24. Cecchi L, D'Amato G, Ayres JG, et al. Projections of the effects of climate change on allergic asthma: the contribution of aerobiology. Allergy 2010;65(9):1073–81.

25. Rogers CA, Wayne PM, Macklin EA, et al. Interaction of the onset of spring and elevated atmospheric CO2 on ragweed (Ambrosia artemisiifolia L.) pollen production. Environ Health Perspect 2006;114(6):865–9.

26. van Vliet AJ, de Groot RS, Bellens Y, et al. The European phenology network. Int J Biometeorol 2003;47(4):202–12.

27. Wayne P, Foster S, Connolly J, et al. Production of allergenic pollen by ragweed (Ambrosia artemisiifolia L.) is increased in CO2-enriched atmospheres. Ann Allergy Asthma Immunol 2002;88(3):279–82.

28. Stach A, Garcia-Mozo H, Prieto-Baena JC, et al. Prevalence of Artemisia species pollinosis in western Poland: impact of climate change on aerobiological trends, 1995-2004. J Investig Allergol Clin Immunol 2007;17(1):39–47.

29. Ahas R, Aasa A. The effects of climate change on the phenology of selected Estonian plant, bird and fish populations. Int J Biometeorol 2006;51(1):17–26.

30. Walther GR, Post E, Convey P, et al. Ecological responses to recent climate change. Nature 2002;416(6879):389–95.

31. Penuelas J, Rutishauser T, Filella I. Ecology. Phenology feedbacks on climate change. Science 2009;324(5929):887–8.

32. Menzel A. Trends in phenological phases in Europe between 1951 and 1996. Int J Biometeorol 2000;44(2):76–81.

33. Picornell A, Buters J, Rojo J, et al. Predicting the start, peak and end of the Betula pollen season in Bavaria, Germany. Sci Total Environ 2019;690:1299–309.

34. Sofiev M, Siljamo P, Ranta H, et al. A numerical model of birch pollen emission and dispersion in the atmosphere. Description of the emission module. Int J Biometeorol 2013;57(1):45–58.

35. Skjoth CA, Sommer J, Stach A, et al. The long-range transport of birch (Betula) pollen from Poland and Germany causes significant pre-season concentrations in Denmark. Clin Exp Allergy 2007;37(8):1204–12.

36. Ziello C, Sparks TH, Estrella N, et al. Changes to airborne pollen counts across Europe. PLoS One 2012;7(4):e34076.

37. Zhang Y, Bielory L, Cai T, et al. Predicting onset and duration of airborne allergenic pollen season in the United States. Atmos Environ (1994) 2015;103:297–306.

38. Ziska LH, Makra L, Harry SK, et al. Temperature-related changes in airborne allergenic pollen abundance and seasonality across the northern hemisphere: a retrospective data analysis. Lancet Planet Health 2019;3(3):e124–31.

39. de Weger LA, Pashley CH, Sikoparija B, et al. The long distance transport of airborne Ambrosia pollen to the UK and the Netherlands from Central and south Europe. Int J Biometeorol 2016;60(12):1829–39.

40. Giejsztowt J, Classen AT, Deslippe JR. Climate change and invasion may synergistically affect native plant reproduction. Ecology 2020;101(1):e02913.

41. Patz JA, Campbell-Lendrum D, Holloway T, et al. Impact of regional climate change on human health. Nature 2005;438(7066):310–7.

42. Bousquet PJ, Burbach G, Heinzerling LM, et al. GA2LEN skin test study III: minimum battery of test inhalent allergens needed in epidemiological studies in patients. Allergy 2009;64(11):1656–62.

43. Dahl R, Andersen PS, Chivato T, et al. National prevalence of respiratory allergic disorders. Respir Med 2004;98(5):398–403.

44. Lemanske RF Jr, Busse WW. Asthma: clinical expression and molecular mechanisms. J Allergy Clin Immunol 2010;125(2 Suppl 2):S95–102.

45. Schatz M, Rosenwasser L. The allergic asthma phenotype. J Allergy Clin Immunol Pract 2014;2(6):645–8 [quiz: 649].

46. Zoratti E, Havstad S, Wegienka G, et al. Differentiating asthma phenotypes in young adults through polyclonal cytokine profiles. Ann Allergy Asthma Immunol 2014;113(1):25–30.

47. Schoos AM, Jelding-Dannemand E, Stokholm J, et al. Single and multiple time-point allergic sensitization during childhood and risk of asthma by age 13. Pediatr Allergy Immunol 2019;30(7):716–23.

48. Taylor PE, Flagan RC, Miguel AG, et al. Birch pollen rupture and the release of aerosols of respirable allergens. Clin Exp Allergy 2004;34(10):1591–6.

49. Spieksma FT, Nikkels AH. Similarity in seasonal appearance between atmospheric birch-pollen grains and allergen in paucimicronic, size-fractionated ambient aerosol. Allergy 1999;54(3):235–41.

50. Renwick DS, Connolly MJ. The relationship between age and bronchial responsiveness: evidence from a population survey. Chest 1999;115(3):660–5.

51. Pyrhonen K, Kulmala P, Nayha S, et al. Diverse age-incidence patterns of atopic sensitization in an unselected Finnish population up to 12 years. Ann Allergy Asthma Immunol 2019;122(5):522–31.e3.

52. Kuparinen A, Katul G, Nathan R, et al. Increases in air temperature can promote wind-driven dispersal and spread of plants. Proc Biol Sci 2009;276(1670): 3081–7.

53. Kim JH, Oh JW, Lee HB, et al. Changes in sensitization rate to weed allergens in children with increased weeds pollen counts in Seoul metropolitan area. J Korean Med Sci 2012;27(4):350–5.

54. Epstein PR. Climate and health. Science 1999;285(5426):347–8.

55. Senechal H, Visez N, Charpin D, et al. A review of the effects of major atmospheric pollutants on pollen grains, pollen content, and allergenicity. ScientificWorldJournal 2015;2015:940243.

56. Schiavoni G, D'Amato G, Afferni C. The dangerous liaison between pollens and pollution in respiratory allergy. Ann Allergy Asthma Immunol 2017;118(3):269–75.

57. Baldacci S, Maio S, Cerrai S, et al. Allergy and asthma: Effects of the exposure to particulate matter and biological allergens. Respir Med 2015;109(9):1089–104.

58. Knox RB, Suphioglu C, Taylor P, et al. Major grass pollen allergen Lol p 1 binds to diesel exhaust particles: implications for asthma and air pollution. Clin Exp Allergy 1997;27(3):246–51.

59. Annesi-Maesano I, Rouve S, Desqueyroux H, et al. Grass pollen counts, air pollution levels and allergic rhinitis severity. Int Arch Allergy Immunol 2012;158(4): 397–404.

60. Villeneuve PJ, Doiron MS, Stieb D, et al. Is outdoor air pollution associated with physician visits for allergic rhinitis among the elderly in Toronto, Canada? Allergy 2006;61(6):750–8.

61. Bohannon J. Climate change. IPCC report lays out options for taming greenhouse gases. Science 2007;316(5826):812–4.

62. D'Amato G, Vitale C, De Martino A, et al. Effects on asthma and respiratory allergy of Climate change and air pollution. Multidiscip Respir Med 2015;10:39.
63. Sheffield PE, Knowlton K, Carr JL, et al. Modeling of regional climate change effects on ground-level ozone and childhood asthma. Am J Prev Med 2011;41(3): 251–7 [quiz: A253].
64. Pollock J, Shi L, Gimbel RW. Outdoor environment and pediatric asthma: an update on the evidence from North America. Can Respir J 2017;2017:8921917.
65. Heguy L, Garneau M, Goldberg MS, et al. Associations between grass and weed pollen and emergency department visits for asthma among children in Montreal. Environ Res 2008;106(2):203–11.
66. D'Amato G, Cecchi L. Effects of climate change on environmental factors in respiratory allergic diseases. Clin Exp Allergy 2008;38(8):1264–74.
67. Choi YJ, Oh HR, Oh JW, et al. Chamber and field studies demonstrate differential amb a 1 contents in common ragweed depending on CO(2) levels. Allergy Asthma Immunol Res 2018;10(3):278–82.
68. Erbas B, Chang JH, Dharmage S, et al. Do levels of airborne grass pollen influence asthma hospital admissions? Clin Exp Allergy 2007;37(11):1641–7.
69. Kim KR, Oh JW, Woo SY, et al. Does the increase in ambient CO2 concentration elevate allergy risks posed by oak pollen? Int J Biometeorol 2018;62(9):1587–94.
70. McMichael AJ. Health consequences of global climate change. J R Soc Med 2001;94(3):111–4.
71. Grewling L, Bogawski P, Kryza M, et al. Concomitant occurrence of anthropogenic air pollutants, mineral dust and fungal spores during long-distance transport of ragweed pollen. Environ Pollut 2019;254(Pt A):112948.
72. Bedard A, Sofiev M, Arnavielhe S, et al. Interactions Between Air Pollution and Pollen Season for Rhinitis Using Mobile Technology: A MASK-POLLAR Study. J Allergy Clin Immunol Pract 2020;8(3):1063–73.e4.

Effect of Climate Change on Allergenic Airborne Pollen in Japan

Reiko Kishikawa, MD, PhD[a],*, Eiko Koto[b]

KEYWORDS

- Allergenic pollen • Climate change • Japanese Cedar • Pollinosis • Immunotherapy

KEY POINTS

- Japanese representative allergenic airborne pollen-related allergic diseases include Cupressaceae in early spring, the birch family and grass in spring and *Artemisia* in autumn.
- The number of Cupressaceae (Japanese Cedar and Cypress) pollen grains is very large.
- An increase in the amount of conifer airborne pollen grains and an earlier start to disperse were observed, related to climate change.
- In addition, an increase in the number and severity of patients with Japanese Cedar pollinosis has been observed.
- Medical pollen information, medication, and sublingual immunotherapy have all been enhanced. Recently, pollen-food allergic syndrome has become of increased interest.

INTRODUCTION

We introduce the important allergenic pollen in Japan according to longitudinal monitoring of airborne pollen all over Japan.

We recognized conifer pollen as the most important because of continuing increase to an already huge number of patients suffering from Japanese Cedar pollinosis.

With a focus on "climate change and allergic diseases," as recommended by Professor Jae-Won Oh, we report long-term survey results of Japanese Cedar (JC) and Cypress family (Cypress) pollen and the related meteorologic conditions in Japan.

Botanically the classification system of Angiosperm Phylogeny Group is gradually taking over from the Copeland/Engler classification system by DNA analysis.[1] In this system, JC belongs to Cupressaceae. However, in Japan, JC is more strongly antigenic than other members of the Cypress family. With this in mind, and due to the

[a] Department of Allergology, National Hospital Organization Fukuoka National Hospital, 4-39-1 Yakatabaru Minami-Ku, Fukuoka 811-1394, Japan; [b] Clinical Research Institute of National Hospital Organization, Fukuoka National Hospital, 4-39-1, Yakatabaru Minami-ku, Fukuoka 811-1394, Japan
* Corresponding author.
E-mail address: kishikawa.reiko.td@mail.hosp.go.jp

Immunol Allergy Clin N Am 41 (2021) 111–125
https://doi.org/10.1016/j.iac.2020.09.005
0889-8561/21/© 2020 Elsevier Inc. All rights reserved.

difference in morphology and term of dispersion, we classified JC separately from other cypresses.

Also, the important allergic pollen grains in Japan have been attracting attention related to pollen-food allergies.

HISTORY

Japanese people had little conception of hay fever (pollinosis) historically. Before World War II, some researchers had reported on and drawn attention to the presence of ragweed hay fever in Japan as being similar to the United States.[2] In 1960, the first case of severe ragweed hay fever was reported with airborne pollen in Tokyo.[2-4] Over the next decade various types of cases such as grass, Japanese hop, mugwort, and occupational hay fever were reported in succession. In 1964, hypersensitivity to JC pollen was reported for the first time.[2,5]

Since the 1970s, the number of patients with JC pollinosis has increased markedly with the huge number of airborne conifer pollen grains dispersing in early spring. This is also influenced by hereditary factors for immune-response and air pollution.[6] In 1986, the Japanese government began to take preventive measures against JC pollinosis and started to investigate JC and Cypress family (Cypress) pollen as an important causative allergen. Planting of JC trees, *Cryptomeria japonica* D. Don trees was promoted throughout broad areas of Japan except in Okinawa Prefecture since the nineteenth century, especially after World War II. The area of national artificial forest more than 31 years old doubled in the 1970s.[7] Generally the amount of JC pollen production is proportional to the area of JC forests aged over 31 years. By 2017, more than 90% of the area was of this age.[8] Planting of trees of the Cypress, Cupressaceae family (mainly *Chamaecyparis obsta*)[9], was also promoted in the same way as JC.

METHOD

We have had to detect allergenic airborne pollen since July 1986. The gravitational method with Durham's sampler has been used.

AIRBORNE POLLEN MONITORING

We have monitored airborne pollen all year round at 26 locations in the Japanese archipelago between the latitudes 30 to 40° north (**Table 1**). At each institute a daily airborne pollen sample was collected by Vaseline-coated glass slides that were fixed in the Durham's sampler, usually exchanged every morning.

The sampling slides were sent to our hospital and pollen number counted per cm² after staining. They were then classified by main pollen grains as a causative agent of pollinosis through the microscope. For the Durham's method, pollen counts were standardized to express them as the number of pollen grains per cm², classifying and summarizing them.[10] For convenience, the number of collected pollen was compiled every 6 months, with the January to June samples classified as spring pollen and the July to December as autumn pollen even if from the same family.

ESTIMATING ALLERGIC CONIFER POLLEN COUNT AND CLIMATIC DATA

In addition, we estimated the pollen count and climatic data close to 9 pollen monitoring locations.[11,12] These are northern regions, Tohoku and Hokuriku (Sendai, Niigata, Toyama); central regions, Kanto, Tokai and Kinki (Sagamihara, Hamamatsu,

Table 1
Geography of pollen monitoring, height of Durham sampler from ground and investigation duration at each institute from north to south of Japan

Institute	City	Latitude	Longitude	Height(m)	Beginning	Duration (Year)
Wagatsuma children clinic	Sapporo	43.05525	141.3455	$16 \rightarrow 7$	Aug 1986	19
Hakodate Hospital	Hakodate	41.78677	140.744	12	Jul. 1995	7
Akita University	Akita	39.74729	140.0834	20	Aug 1986	6
West Taga Chest Hospital	Sendai	38.25416	140.8414	12	Aug. 1986	4
Tohoku University	Sendai	38.25416	140.8414	20	Jul. 1986	31
Fukushima Chest Hospital	Fukushima	37.74891	140.37	8	Mar. 1990	2
Fujisaki Clinic	Niigata	37.92084	139.0533	3	Jan. 1987	29
Tsukioka Clinic	Niigata	37.92084	139.0533	8	Jul. 1986	21
Toyama University	Toyama	36.69124	137.2201	20	Jul. 1986	27
Tokyo Hospital	Kiyose	35.76606	139.506	16	Jul. 1986	6
Sato Clinic	Takasaki	36.32537	139.0162	6	Jan. 1998	21
NHO Sagamihara Hospital	Sagamihara	35.48806	139.1608	20	Oct1986	28
Tokai Pollinosis Institute	Hamamatsu	35.68907	139.7874	$37 \rightarrow 6$	Jul. 1986	33
NHO Mie Hospital	Tsu	34.71911	136.5168	8	Jul. 1986	32
Osaka Medical University	Osaka	34.70251	135.4965	40	May. 1986	7
Wakayama Redcross Hospital	Wakayama	34.22198	135.1661	$16 \rightarrow 18$	Jan. 1987	31
Matsue Chest Hospital	Matsue	35.46905	133.0616	8	Sep. 1986	18
East Kochi Chest Hospital	Kochi	33.55201	133.5383	10	Jan. 1987	15
Kyushu University	Fukuoka	33.57979	130.4024	21	Jul. 1986	28
NHO Fukuoka Hospital	Fukuoka	33.57979	130.4024	16	Jul. 1986	33
Nagasaki University	Nagasaki	32.76542	129.8663	16	Jul. 1986	29
Kumamoto University	Kumamoto	32.78852	130.7149	40	Jul. 1986	29
Fujimoto-Hayasuzu Hospital	Miyakonojo	35.66897	139.477	21	Jul. 1986	20
Miyazaki University	Miyazaki	31.90738	131.5525	5	Jul. 1986	29
Hokusatsu Hospital	Oguchi	32.03073	130.5871	5	Jul. 1986	19
Kumage Branch Office	Yakushima	30.25635	130.5028	8	Jan. 1998	21

Table 1 shows the geographic location of each pollen monitoring institute, the height of the sampler from the ground, and pollen investigation duration from north to south of Japan.

Tsu, Wakayama); and in the south-west, Kyushu district (Fukuoka, Kumamoto) as shown in **Table 2**. We referred to the annual change in monthly mean temperature using the Japan Weather Association Home Page database. We have estimated annual total pollen counts and yearly starting day of JC pollen dispersal with climatic conditions statistically. Stata (StateCorp LLC, USA/ Lightstone Co. LTD, Tokyo, Japan) was used for statistical analysis.

RESULTS
Representative Airborne Pollen as Allergenic Agent

Tree pollen[12]: As **Fig. 1** shows, tree total pollen count at each location was averaging 889 ~ 13,116 pollen grains per year. JC pollen was most common, at 40%, with the Cypress family next at approximately 20%, together more than 60% of pollen in the sample. These pollen counts increased with the annual fluctuation. In Hokkaido, the prevalence of birch family pollen in the count was larger.

Herbaceous pollen[13]: Total herbaceous pollen counts at each location were extremely small compared with tree pollen, averaging 73 ~ 650 pollen grains (**Fig. 2**). The Sagamihara location had the highest count. Spring grass pollen gave the largest count, at 30% of the total collected. *Artemisia* pollen is scarce, but it is found across the country, with 6 ~ 40 pollen count per cm^2 in autumn. *Ambrosia* was less in evidence than *Artemisia* except in Sagamihara and Miyazaki (333,88).

Annual Conifer Pollen Grains Count and Climate Change

Fig. 3 shows the annual fluctuation of the conifer pollen counts (JC, Cypress) at the 9 locations in Japan (see **Table 2**). Each vertical line shows pollen counts per cm^2 per year and horizontal line shows year. We did not express pollen counts logarithmically because it is difficult to show the annual fluctuation visually. JC pollen counts are indicated by the blue bar and Cypress by the red. Each dotted line shows the approximation line. Both pollen counts have been increasing gradually over time. The pollen counts per cm^2/year are different for each location. In Sagamihara, the highest JC pollen count was observed. In Tohoku, Cypress pollen counts were lower than in other regions, and in Kyushu, Cypress pollen counts have increased.

Table 2
The locations of airborne pollen monitoring by Durham's Sampler over a long period. There are 9 institutions in Sendai, Niigata, Toyama, Sagamihara, Hamamatsu, Tsu, Wakayama, Fukuoka, and Kumamoto

NO	City	District	Institute	Latitude	Longitude	Survey Period (year)
1	Sendai	Tohoku	Tohoku University	38.25416	140.8414	31
2	Niigata	Hokuriku	Fujisaki Clinic	37.92084	139.0533	29
3	Toyama	Hokuriku	Toyama University	36.69124	137.2201	27
4	Sagamihara	Kanto	NHO Sagamihara Hospital	35.48806	139.1608	28
5	Hamamatsu	Tokai	Tokai Pollinosis Institute	35.68907	139.7874	33
6	Tsu	Kinki	NHO Mie Hospital	34.71911	136.5168	32
7	Wakayama	Kinki	Wakayama Red cross Hospital	34.22198	135.1661	31
8	Fukuoka	Kyushu	NHO Fukuoka Hospital	33.57979	130.4024	33
9	Kumamoto	Kyushu	Kumamoto University	32.78852	130.7149	29

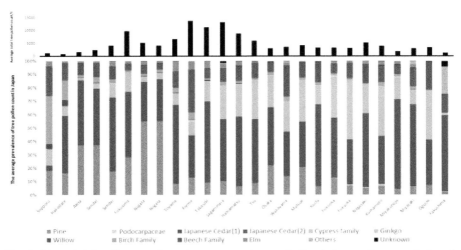

Fig. 1. Mean total pollen counts and mean prevalence of allergic tree pollen count at each location from Sapporo to Yakushima. The upper histogram shows mean total pollen counts. The Kiyose and Sagaminara locations had the highest counts. Each bar chart shows mean prevalence of pollen count. At all locations with the exception of Sapporo city, JC and Cypress family pollen were the most prevalent pollen at approximately 60% of the total. In Sapporo, the prevalence of birch pollen count was greater.

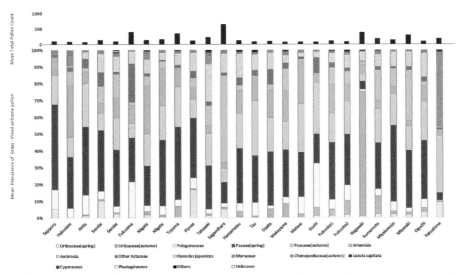

Fig. 2. Mean total pollen counts and mean prevalence of allergic herbaceous pollen counts at each location from Sapporo to Yakushima. The upper histogram shows mean total pollen counts. The Sagaminara location had the greatest count. The lower bar chart shows mean prevalence of pollen counts at each location. The red element shows grass (Poaceae) pollen in spring at each location: it was the largest element with a mean of 30%. Ambrosia in Sagamihara and Urticaceae in Nagasaki stood out in particular.

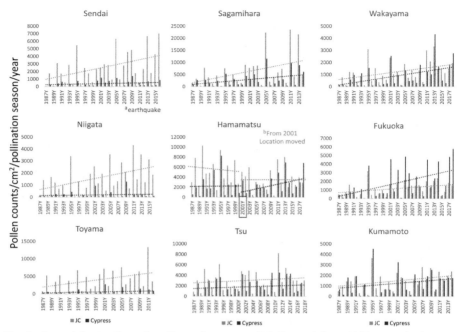

Fig. 3. Annual fluctuation of conifer pollen counts (JC, Cypress) from 1987 to, at the longest 2018, at 9 locations in Japan. Each vertical line shows pollen counts and the horizontal line shows the year. Both pollen counts have shown remarkable annual fluctuation and totals have been increasing gradually. In Sagamihara, the highest JC pollen count was observed. [a] The East of Japan Earthquake March 11, 2011. [b] In Hamamatsu the monitoring location was moved in 2001.

Fig. 4 shows the annual change in mean temperature at the 9 cities in July and August when JC and Cypress male flower buds are growing. Each vertical line shows mean monthly temperature and the horizontal line shows year and the dotted line shows the approximation. The monthly mean temperatures rise in all regions without exception.

Table 1 shows the correlation between the mean temperature in summer and the next year's annual total pollen count. There are significant positive correlations between the annual summer mean temperature and the next year's total pollen counts of JC and Cypress especially the counts in July ($P<.05$ to $<.0001$). The higher the summer temperature, the more significantly conifer rose in these pollen counts.

Annual Japanese Cedar Pollination Starting Day and Climate Change

Fig. 5 shows the annual change of starting day in JC pollination. Each vertical line shows days since January 1, and each horizontal line shows the year.

The dotted line shows the approximate. The starting day is earlier in Tohoku (Sendai, Niigata), Hokuriku (Toyama), and later in Kanto (Sagamihara), Tokai (Hamamatsu), and Kinki (Tsu, Wakayama) regions. In Kyushu districts (Fukuoka, Kumamoto), they are almost static.

Fig. 6 shows the annual change of monthly mean temperature of January and February just before and after the JC pollination season. Each vertical line shows

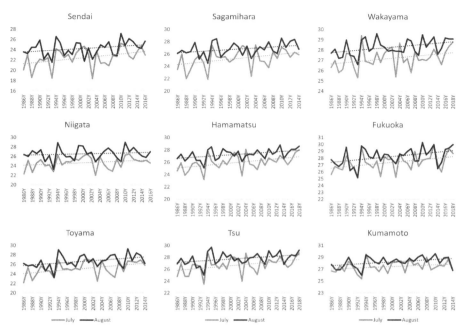

Fig. 4. Annual change of mean temperature in July and August from 1986 to, at latest, 2018 in Japan. In summer, the JC and Cypress male flower bud forms. The vertical line shows mean monthly temperature and horizontal line shows year, and the dotted line shows the approximation. In July and August the monthly mean temperatures are rising of all areas without exception.

monthly mean temperature and the horizontal line shows the year. There has been a gradual fall in January and rise in February, although the change range is very small in Hokuriku and there is almost no change in Tohoku regions.

Tables 3 and **4** show the correlation between the start day of JC pollination and the mean temperature in January (blue line) and February (red line) when the JC pollen grains are nearly beginning to disperse. In February, we found a significantly strong negative correlation between the starting day and mean temperature ($P = .05$ to $P<.0001$), in Sendai, Niigata, and Toyama, north of Japan. In January there are weak negative significant correlations in Sagamihara, Hamamatsu, and Tsu ($P = .03$ to $P = .003$). Due to winter climate change over 30 years, the starting day has become earlier in northern regions, and later in central Japan.

DISCUSSION

In 1986, we started these investigations at 47 institutes, one in each prefecture in Japan, and 26 institutions have continued to investigate for more than 2 years (see **Table 1**). For the first 9 years, we investigated using a research fund of the Ministry of Health.[14] After that, we continued monitoring airborne pollen on a Voluntary basis.

The Appearance of Pollen-Food Allergic Syndrome/Oral Allergic Syndrome

In our country, airborne pollen of the JC and Cypress, the birch family, grass in spring, *Artemisia* and *Ambrosia* in autumn are representative pollens causing allergic diseases.

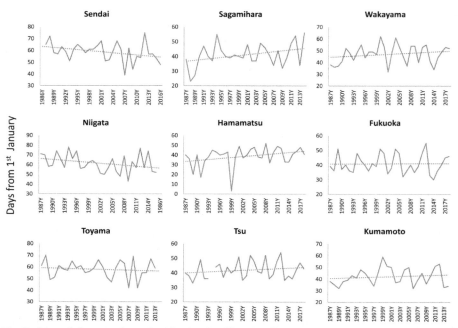

Fig. 5. Annual change of starting day in JC pollination from 1987 to, at the latest, 2018. Each vertical line shows days from January 1 and the horizontal line shows year. The start day, counting from January 1, is earlier in Tohoku (Sendai, Niigata), Hokuriku (Toyama) district, and later in Kanto (Sagamihara), Tokai (Hamamatsu) and Kinki (Tsu, Wakayama) districts. In Kyushu districts (Fukuoka, Kumamoto) it is static.

The amount of JC and Cypress pollen is very large. People with pollen allergies have rhinoconjunctivitis mainly in each pollination season with allergic pharyngitis, asthma, and allergic dermatitis exacerbation. However, from approximately 2000, rose family fruit food allergy due to the birch pollen antigen in Hokkaido[15] was reported and the number of patients with pollen-food allergic syndrome (PFAS) has increased with increasing birch family pollen production.[16] In Kanto region and West Japan also, alder and mugwort PFAS with pollinosis has been reported.[17,18] In Kyushu, trees of alder pollen (from the birch family) are counted in very small numbers. But adult and infant patients with rose family fruit food allergy[19] are consulted. In Kyushu there are trees of the beech family such as oak ,and the pollen production from these is increasing.[20] There is cross-reactivity between the beech and birch family pollen antigen[21] but this is not yet proven to be related to PFAS/oral allergic syndrome (OAS).[22] However, this suggests that we need to carefully examine the rhinoconjuctivitis and PFAS/OAS related to these possibly problematic trees and herbaceous pollen. The number of articles on PFAS has increased from approximately 2000, and the review articles reported until then that the main symptoms were mainly rhinoconjunctivitis and respiratory in Europe and the United States.[23,24] We believe the number of PFAS patients has increased[25] with the increase in pollen antigen related with climate change.

Japanese Cedar Pollinosis Has Been the Most Important for a Long Time

Japan has extensive forests, with 70% total coverage of the country as a whole. The conifer pollen grain continued to be the most important allergic causative agents.

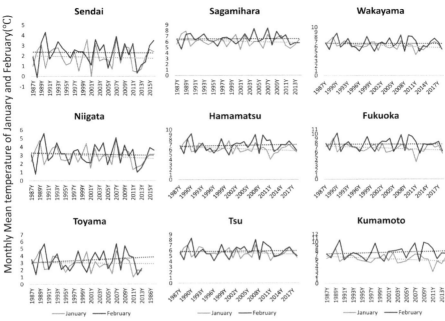

Fig. 6. The annual change of monthly mean temperature of January and February from 1986 to, at latest, 2018. Each vertical line shows monthly mean temperature and horizontal line shows year. The dotted line shows the approximation. It gradually falls in January (*blue line*) and rises in February (*red line*), although the change range is very small in Hokuriku and there is almost no change in Tohoku region.

National JC forests are aging because they are no longer being used for timber. Cypress pollen has strong cross-reactivity to JC. Many patients with allergy to conifer have exacerbated symptoms every spring. In 1998, the prevalence of JC pollinosis was 16% on average but rose to 26.5% on average, with a particular increase in infants with JC pollinosis, by 2008.[26]

Gravitational Monitoring Is Primitive but Adequate for Pollen Information

Durham's sampler was a technically simple method used by our predecessors, as it was immediately available and easy applicable by allergy professional clinicians in the 1960s.[27] Durham's sampler has become the most popular in Japan. This technique is now almost outdated but is still suited to gathering daily information about huge numbers of pollen grains, for the medical benefit of patients with pollinosis. We reported a strong positive correlation between Durham's and volumetric sampler (Burkard's sampler) conifer pollen counting in 2009.[28] We now have more than 400 locations observing JC and Cypress pollen count to gather nationwide pollen information.

Meteorologic Conditions Affect Conifer Pollen Production

JC and Cypress pollen production is related to higher temperatures and lower humidity conditions in the previous summer, when male flower formed. The start of pollination has been influenced by meteorologic conditions around the time of male flower maturation. Male flower bud formation and dispersal of pollen depends on weather

Table 3
Correlation between total pollen counts of conifer pollen from 1987 to, at latest, 2018 and the previous year's July and August mean temperature in male flower bud formation

City	Duration (Y)	July		August	
Japanese Cedar					
Sendai	n = 30	r = 0.397	P<.05	r = 0.145	P = .443
Niigata	n = 30	r = 0.639	P<.001	r = 0.452	P<.05
Toyama	n = 26	r = 0.652	P<.001	r = 0.639	P<.001
Sagamihara	n = 28	r = 0.613	P<.001	r = 0.499	P<.01
Hamamatsu	n = 32	r = 0.390	P<.05	NS	
Tsu	n = 31	r = 0.696	P<.0001	NS	
Wakayama	n = 32	r = 0.630	P<.001	r = 0.491	P<.01
Fukuoka	n = 32	r = 0.736	P<.0001	r = 0.668	P<.0001
Kumamoto	n = 28	r = 0.737	P<.0001	r = 0.638	P<.001
Cypress family					
Sendai	n = 30	r = 0.558	P = .0014	NS	
Niigata	n = 30	r = 0.718	P<.0001	r = 0.414	P<.05
Toyama	n = 26	r = 0.694	P<.0001	r = 0.546	P<.01
Sagamihara	n = 28	r = 0.598	P<.001	r = 0.475	P<.05
Hamamatsu	n = 32	r = 0.539	P<.01	r = 0.446	P<.05
Tsu	n = 31	r = 0.597	P<.001	r = 0.390	P<.05
Wakayama	n = 32	r = 0.627	P<.001	r = 0.414	P<.05
Fukuoka	n = 32	r = 0.676	P<.0001	r = 0.650	P<.0001
Kumamoto	n = 28	r = 0.6S6	P<.001	r = 0.505	P<.01

Spearman's rank correlation coefficient.
Generally production of conifer pollen correlates with the previous summer's climate condition with the temperature and humidity. There are significant positive correlations between the annual summer mean temperature and the following year's total pollen counts especially the July temperature
Abbreviation: NS, not significant.

conditions and geographic features. We estimated the regional pollen data under some meteorologic conditions and hope to predict these pollen dispersal trends in coming years as the climate changes.

Annual Pollen Counting and Climate Change

As **Fig. 3** shows, for both of pollen, annual fluctuation has been measured in each location. In Sagamihara the highest JC pollen count was observed, but fewer than 1000 to more than 20,000 pollen grains per cm^2/season were counted. Everywhere pollen counting has seen remarkable annual fluctuations. In Tohoku, Cypress pollen counts were less than that of other regions. In Kyushu, Cypress pollen counts have increased more than those of JC. Monthly mean temperatures are going to rise in all areas. There is a significant positive correlation between the annual summer mean temperature and the next year's total pollen counts especially in July when the male flower bud is formatted. The higher the summer temperature, the more these conifer pollen counts increase. The production of both types of pollen grains are higher in the Kanto and Tokai regions where a large percentage of the population lives. In those regions exposed to large amounts of pollen antigen, there are many patients

Table 4
Correlation between starting day of Japanese Cedar pollination and mean temperature near pollinated season from 1987 to, at latest, 2018

City	Years	January Average Temperature		February Average Temperature	
Sendai	30	r = −0.500	P = .005	r = −0.774	P<.0001
Niigata	30	NS		r = −0.645	P = .0001
Toya ma	27	NS		r = −0.827	P<.0001
Sagamihara	28	r = −0.549	P = .003	NS	
Hamamatsu	32	r = −0.373	P = .036	NS	
Tsu	31	r = −0.414	P = .021	NS	
Wakayama	32	r = −0.397	P = .025	NS	
Fukuoka	32	NS		NS	
Kumamoto	28	NS		NS	

Spearman's rank correlation coefficient.
   Table 4 shows the correlation between starting day of JC pollination and the mean temperature in January and February when the JC pollen grains are nearly beginning to disperse. In February we found significant negative correlation between the starting day and winter mean temperature.
   Abbreviation: NS, not significant.

with serious rhinoconjunctivitis, including systemic allergic symptoms and related food allergies such as PFAS/OAS.[29–31]

Annual Starting Day of Japanese Cedar Pollen Dispersing and Climate Change

It is important to know the starting date of pollination before the season for successful treatment. Currently the prediction of the start of JC pollen dispersal everywhere is an essential measure for treating JC pollinosis.

   The start day is earlier in the north of Japan, and later in central Japan where there is a huge dispersal of pollen. We believe that JC pollination season will commence at almost the same time at each region in the near future.

   JC male flowers need low temperatures to produce dormancy in winter followed by higher temperature to trigger pollination after the dormancy period. We found significant negative correlation between the start day of pollination and winter mean temperature. This is especially clear in the north of Japan in February.

   Since approximately 1994, a little JC pollen dispersion has been monitored from October to December,[32] and the number of pollen grains is increasing. We believe this may be one of the effects of climate change.

Social and Medical Background of Japanese Cedar Pollinosis Treatment

The total cost of treatment of patients with JC pollinosis and associated diseases is $3 billion.[33] For this reason, the Japanese government has worked to find preventive measures. In the medical and health welfare fields there is continuous research into allergy and immunology including JC pollinosis. In addition, the Forest Agency and the Ministry of Environment have many projects, including nonproductive pollen cedar bleeding,[34] promoting of comfortable forest without JC/Cypress around big cities, a nationwide information network, and the precise prediction of pollen dispersal. We now have a full pollen network system by Durham's Sampler. Real-time auto monitor for selected pollen grains has been developed over the past decade in the Ministry of Environment. However, there are many problems in making a useful, popular, and long-lasting pollen information and forecast system to prevent pollinosis exacerbation. On the other hand, sublingual immunotherapy of JC has been developed and the therapeutic effect was seen.[35,36] This method is suitable for all patients in all age groups. In addition, improved medication has been introduced every year adding to treatment of pollinosis guidelines.[26] Continuous efforts to overcome pollinosis in all generations are still ongoing in our country.

Perspectives and Conclusion

In Japan, allergenic conifer pollen counts have been increasing because areas with aged conifer plantations and also through the effects of climate change over 30 years. We need to know the allergenic pollen grains and to apply the results to deal with it. PFAS due to allergenic pollen is likely to increase in all generations.

Clinics care points

- Antigen avoidance: Daily pollen forecast is useful. In addition, we must understand the types of important pollen antigens and the pollination season.

- Early treatment for successful treatment: we must obtain information for predicting the start of cedar pollen dispersal and start treatment before dispersal.

- We should continue treatment during the dispersal period to prevent the exacerbation and aggravation of comorbidities such as bronchial asthma, pollen dermatitis, and PFAS.

ACKNOWLEDGMENTS

The authors thank many collaborators and around people related these study for a long time following Sendai (Tohoku University Otolaryngology Laboratory), Niigata (Fujisaki Clinic, Tsukioka Clinic), Toyama (Toyama University), Takasaki (Sato Kei Clinic), Sagamihara (NHO Sagamihara Hospital), Hamamatsu (Tokai Pollinosis Institute), Tsu (NHO Mie Hospital), Wakayama (Wakayama Red Cross Hosp.), Fukuoka (Kyushu University), Kumamoto (Kumamoto University), Miyazaki (Miyazaki University) and Yakushima (Kagoshima University, The Foresty Agency), and Japan Weather Support Center, Environmental Ministry, Fukuoka Prefecture Medical Association, Japan Medical University, Oita University. We appreciate the Ministry of Health and Welfare funds from 1986 to 1995 for monitoring airborne pollen survey.

Also the authors thank to Honor director of our hospital the late Hitoshi Nagano, Sankei Nishima, MD, PhD, the late Mitue Katuta, MD, PhD, Yoshinori Wagatsuma, MD, PhD (Wagatsuma chirdren clinic), the late Takao Shida, MD, PhD (Sagamihara National Hospital), Honor Professor Estelle Levetin (The University of Tulsa, Tulsa, Oklahoma), Honor Professor Randy Goldberm, Associate Professor Termi M. Horiuti and Edward Brooks (University of Texas Medical Branch, USA), Honor Professor Jean Emberlin (Worcester University, UK).

Moreover, the authors thank the respected collaborators for about 30 years, Norio Sahashi, PhD, Nobuo Soh, MD, PhD, Toshitaka Yokoyama, PhD, Tadao Enomoto, MD, PhD, Toru Imai, MD, PhD, Koji Murayama, PhD, Atsushi Usami, MD, PhD, Hidetoyo Teranishi, MD, PhD, Yoko Fujisaki, MD, PhD, Akemi Ishii, Secretary, and the late Motoo Suzuki, PhD (NPO Pollen Information Association), Akemi Saito, PhD, Yuma Fukutomi, MD, PhD, Masami Taniguchi, MD, PhD (NHO Sagamihara National Hospital), Yasuhiro Samjima, MD, PhD (Kumamoto University), Takao Fujisawa, MD, PhD (NHO Mie National Hospital), Chie Oshikawa, MD, PhD, Akiko Sugiyama, MD, Koki Okabe, MD, Takehito Fukushima, MD, PhD, Kaoru Kojima, Tec, Makiko Oda, Tec,

Terufumi Shimoda, MD, PhD, Satoshi Honjo, MD, PhD, Makoto Yoshida, MD, PhD, and Tomoaki Iwanaga, MD, PhD (NHO Fukuoka National Hospital).
Thank you for English Proofreading, Nick May.

REFERENCES

1. Yonekura K, Murata H, supervisor. Higher plant classification Scheme. Tokyo (Japan): Hokuryukan; 2010. p. 13–28, 34–6. [in Japanese].
2. Ishizaki T. History a University of Texas Medical Branch nd definition of hay fever. In: Ishizaki T, editor. Pollen allergy of Circumstance and treatment. Tokyo (Japan): Hokuryukan; 1979. p. 1–7 [in Japanese].
3. Araki H. Studies on Pollinosis 1. Pollen Survey in Tokyo its Neighboring District. Arerugi 1960;9:648–55 [in Japanese].
4. Araki H. Studies on Pollinosis II.Sensitization with pollen in Japan. Arerugi 1961; 10:354–70 [in Japanese].
5. Saito Y, Horiguchi S. Japanese Cedar pollinosis in Nikko Japan. Arerugi 1964;13: 16–8 [in Japanese].
6. Ishizaki T, Koizumi K, Ikemori R, et al. Studies of prevalence of Japanese cedar pollinosis among the residents in a densely cultivated area. Ann Allergy 1987;58: 265–70.
7. Yokoyama T, Kanazasi T. Annual change in the area of Japanese Cedar forest as a source of allergic pollen. In: Muranaka M, Taniguchi K, editors. Immune- goblin E antibody and environmental factors. Tokyo: Medical Tribune; 1990. p. 67–78 [in Japanese].
8. Yokoyama T. A bite note of Japanese Cedar pollinosis,p6. Available at: http://www.tokyo-eiken.go.jp/kj_kankyo/kafun/hitokuti/.
9. Makino T, Honda S, editors. Makino's illustrated flora in colour. Tokyo: Hokuryu-kan; 1982. p. 810.
10. Sahashi N, Nishima S, Kishikawa R, et al. Standardization of procedures for atmo-spheric pollen counts and pollen forecast in Japan. Jpn J Palynol 1993;39: 129–34 [in Japanese].
11. Kishikawa R, Oshikawa C, Koto E, et al. Longitudinal investigation on allergenic conifer pollen in japan for successful prevention and treatment against Japanese Cedar Pollinosis. Expert Opin Environ Biol 2016;5:2.
12. Kishikawa R, Koto E, Oshikawa C, et al. Longitudinal monitoring of tree airborne pollen in Japan- regional distribution and annual change of important allergenic tree pollen. Arerugi 2017;66:97–111.
13. Kishikawa R, Koto E, Oshikawa C, et al. Long-term results of airborne pollen sur-veys in the Japanese archiago from the perspective of pollen antigen. – regional and annual variation of important herbaceous pollen antigen in Japan-. Arerugi 2019;68:1221–38 [in Japanese].
14. Nishima S, Okuda M, Shida T, et al. Edi: Ministry of Health and Welfare pollen research Group, pollen survey in the Japanese Islands data Base. Tokyo: Kyowa-kikaku; 2000. p. 1–261.
15. Asakura K, Honnma A, Yamasaki T, et al. Relationships between oral allergy syn-drome and sensitization to pollen antigen, especially to Mugwort. Arerugi 2006; 55:811–9.
16. Kobayasi T, Takeuchi S, Yasaka M. Trends in annual counts of *Betula* pollen from six cities in Hokkaido. Jpn J Palynol 2013;59:59–67 [in Japanese].

17. Maeda N, Inomata N, Morita A, et al. Correlation of oral allergy syndrome due to plant-derived foods with pollen sensitization in Japan. Ann Allergy Asthma Immunol 2010;104:205–10.
18. Adachi A, Horikawa T. Local differences of oral allergy syndrome with pollinosis: a comparison between Hanshinkan and Higashiharima in Southhyogo. Arerugi 2006;55:811–9.
19. Masumoto N, Teduka J, Nanishi M, et al. Pollen food allergy syndrome in five-year-old boy after moving house at the foot of the mountain: a case report. Arerugi 2018;67:1027–32 [in Japanese].
20. Kishikawa R, Yokoyama T, Sahashi N, et al. Effect of climate change on Fagaceaec airborne pollen in Japan as allergic causative agent associated with food allergy. J Geogr Nat Disast 2016;6:3.
21. Koya K. A study on pollinosis : III. The significance of oak (genus *Quercus*) in pollinosis. Arerugi 1970;19(918–30):933–93 [in Japanese].
22. ALLERGEN NOMENCLATURE, WHO/IUIS Allergen Nomenclature Sub-Committee ,WHO/IUIS Allergen Nomenclature Home Page. Available at: http://www.allergen.org/.
23. Carlson G, Coop C. Pollen food allergy syndrome (PFAS): A review of current available literature. Ann Allergy Asthma Immunol 2019;123:359–65.
24. D'Amato G, Spieksma F, Liccardi G, et al. Pollen-related allergy in Europe. Allergy 1998;53:567–78.
25. Lee SC, Kim SR, Park KH, et al. Clinical features and culprit food allergens of Korean adult food allergy patients: a cross-sectional single-institute study. Allergy Asthma Immunol Res 2019;11:723–35.
26. Committee on Practical guidelines for the Management of Allergic Rhinitis in Japan: Epidemiology of Japanese cedar pollinosis in Japan, practical guidelines for the management of allergic rhinitis in Japan. Tokyo: Life Science; 2015. p. 7–13 [in Japanese].
27. Saito A, Murakami A, Fukutomi Y, et al. Fifty-year record of airborne pollen in Sagamihara, Japan. Jpn J Palynol 2017;62:75–85.
28. Kishikawa R, Sahashi N, Saito A, et al. Japanese Cedar airborne pollen monitoring by Durham's and Burkard Samplers in Japan- Estimation of the usefulness of Durham's Sampler on Japanese Cedar pollinosis. Glob Environ Res 2009;13: 55–61.
29. Inuo C, Kondo Y, Tanaka K, et al. Japanese cedar pollen-based subcutaneous immunotherapy decreases tomato fruit-specific basophil activation. Int Arch Allergy Immunol 2015;167:137–45.
30. Bonds R, Sharma GS, Kondo Y, et al. Pollen food allergy syndrome to tomato in mountain cedar pollen hypersensitivity. Mol Immunol 2019;111:83–6.
31. Sénéchal H, Keykhosravi S, Couderc R, et al. Pollen/fruit syndrome: clinical relevance of the cypress pollen allergenic gibberellin-regulated protein. Allergy Asthma Immunol Res 2019;11:143–51.
32. Taira H, Teranishi H, Kenda Y. Sugi (*Cryptomeria japonica* D. Don) pollen scattering out of season. Arerugi 1992;41:1466–71 [in Japanese].
33. Ogino S. Loss of work productivity in patients with Japanese Cedar pollinosis. Jpn J Occup Environ Allergol 2015;22:25–31 [in Japanese].
34. Saito M, Goto S. Doubling the production of male sterile Japanese cedar (*Cryptomeria japonica* D. Don) seedlings by application of micro-cutting technique. Jpn J FGTB (Forest Genetics and Tree Breeding) 2019;8:1–7 [in Japanese].

35. Yuta A, Ogihara H, Miyamoto Y, et al. The enhanced clinical efficacy by treated years and the sustained efficacy after treatment of sublingual immunotherapy for Japanese cedar pollinosis]. Arerugi 2010;59:1552–61 [in Japanese].
36. Okamoto Y, Okubo K, Yonekura S, et al. Efficacy and safety of sublingual immunotherapy for two seasons in patients with Japanese cedar pollinosis. Int Arch Allergy Immunol 2015;166:177–88.

Forecast for Pollen Allergy
A Review from Field Observation to Modeling and Services in Korea

Kyu Rang Kim, PhD[a],*, Mae Ja Han, MS[b], Jae-Won Oh, MD, PhD[c,d]

KEYWORDS

- Pollen • Observation • Calendar • Forecast • Allergy risks • Climate change

KEY POINTS

- Daily pollen monitoring helps understanding regional differences and long-term changes in pollen allergy risks.
- Pollen risks forecasts of 2 to 3 days are possible using daily forecasts and the relationship between daily pollen concentration and weather conditions.
- Increasing temperature and CO_2 concentration during the climate change will elevate the risks by the pollen allergy in the future.

INTRODUCTION

It is well established that the severity of allergic symptoms is related to airborne pollen concentration.[1–8] Forecast services for pollen-related allergy risk are provided in many countries.[9–12] The basic data and models of such services are pollen observation and modeling.[13–29] The Korea Meteorological Administration (KMA) operates a daily pollen-monitoring network, develops forecast models, and provides daily pollen forecast.[30–32] The major efforts exerted during the last 20+ years for pollen forecast in Korea are summarized in this review to provide the readers with insight on forecast systems and their critical components of observation, modeling, and service.

OBSERVATION

For the prediction of allergy risks by pollen, pollen concentration has long been observed at many places worldwide. The KMA along with the Korean Academy of

[a] High Impact Weather Research Department, National Institute of Meteorological Sciences, 7 Jukheon-gil, Gangneung-si, Gangwon-do 25457, Republic of Korea; [b] High Impact Weather Research Department, National Institute of Meteorological Sciences, 153 Gyeongchun-ro, Guri 11923, Republic of Korea; [c] Department of Pediatrics, Hanyang University Guri Hospital, 153 Gyeongchun-ro, Guri 11923, Republic of Korea; [d] Hanyang University College of Medicine, Seoul, Republic of Korea
* Corresponding author.
E-mail address: krk9@kma.go.kr

Immunol Allergy Clin N Am 41 (2021) 127–141
https://doi.org/10.1016/j.iac.2020.09.011
0889-8561/21/© 2020 Elsevier Inc. All rights reserved.

Pediatric Allergy and Respiratory Disease (KAPARD) established the national pollen observational network in Korea in 1997. As of 2020, the network is composed of 12 stations with Burkard traps. Using 7-day recording drums and an optical microscope, daily pollen concentrations of all species are collected, identified, and counted in each site, every week (**Fig. 1**).[33]

- Pros: It constitutes real observational data, on which both model development and validation are based. In other words, all diagnostic and forecasting models are basically developed using these data.
- Cons: The entire process needs much effort and takes a long time from observation to identification resulting in at least 7 days, or more, delay. It is a site-specific observation and cannot fully represent the spatial distribution of pollen species and counts.

POLLEN CALENDAR

Pollen season, a specific time period with many region-specific pollen grains in the air, is a yearly phenomenon. Pollen calendar, which indicates the region, period, and species of abundant pollen, is developed based on this recurrence.

The methods can be simply temporal averaging or statistical derivation from a probability density function.

The first pollen calendar in Korea was developed in 2004 using observational data gathered from 1997 to 2002. It presented national average pollen seasons of 21 species.[34] After 10 years of observation, regional pollen characteristics were analyzed. Moreover, revised pollen calendars were developed.[34,35] The pollen calendar shows major pollen species and region seasons. Although pollen species in Korea are largely similar around the country, there are regional differences both in representative species and their peak concentrations. The 3 data points of each month are selected out of 10-day running averages from 6 observational stations (Seoul, Busan, Daegu, Gwangju, Gangneung, and Jeju). Several key points are identified from the calendar.

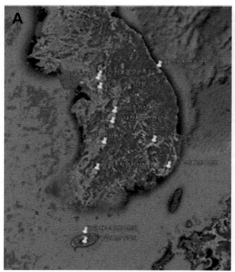 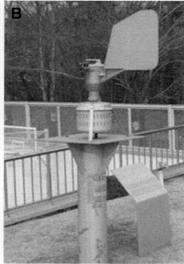

Fig. 1. (*A*) Pollen observation network in Korea and (*B*) Burkard pollen trap. (*From* Google Maps. Available at: https://www.google.com/maps/ Accessed: 2020; with permission.)

Pine is the most abundant species at most stations; although, it presents low allergenicity. Japanese cedar is the most abundant species in Jeju. Warmer southern stations have earlier pollen seasons than northern ones. The pollen species with high allergenicity and large extent are oak and Japanese hop. In the pollen calendar, warning levels of pollen allergenicity are standardized for trees, grasses, and weeds. Its Impacts on Korean patients could have been inconsistent, because the levels were adapted from the US standard[36] without a rigorous statistical analysis.

As the observation continues after the development of the pollen calendar based on the first 10 years of observation, there are accumulated changes in vegetation distribution and land use as well as regional climate. The pollen calendar must reflect these changes using the newly observed data. In addition to the original 6 stations, 2 more were added (Jeonju and Daejeon) to fully use all data gathered from 2007 to 2017. The daily mean of observed data during the 11 years were smoothed using probability density functions, which were fitted using Julian day as X (independent variable) and pollen concentration as Y (dependent variable) for individual species and stations. The risk benchmarks according to pollen concentration were also determined using the fitted probability distribution for each pollen species. Consistent benchmarks are needed due to the necessity of magnitude comparison regarding the concentrations across the nation despite its high spatial variability. The highest magnitudes among the studied stations in South Korea were considered the benchmark concentrations for each pollen species. The 4 levels in the benchmarks are defined as low (0%–50%), moderate (51%–75%), high (76%–87.5%), and very high (87.6%–100%) in **Table 1**. The actual risk level values were determined from the cumulative distribution curves of the fitted distribution. The periods of yearly cumulative pollen, less than 2.5% or more than 97.5%, were removed from the calendar to prevent unnecessary lengthening of the pollen season. In this way, the pollen risk information for each city was consistently developed and delivered. The revised calendar shows regional risks more clearly with continuous pollen periods in contrast to the older version.[37] It only has one benchmark for a pollen species so that one can compare pollen risks

Table 1
Benchmarks of pollen concentration levels used in the pollen calendar of Korean cities

Allergenic Pollens	Concentration Levels			
	Low	Moderate	High	Very High
Alder	0–6	7–27	28–60	≥61
Japanese cedar	0–12	13–54	55–127	≥128
Birch	0–6	7–15	16–27	≥28
Hazelnut	0–3	4–9	10–15	≥16
Oak	0–14	15–56	57–133	≥134
Elm	0–5	6–15	16–30	≥31
Pine	0–6	7–33	34–86	≥87
Ginkgo	0–16	17–67	68–152	≥153
Chestnut	0–5	6–17	18–33	≥34
Grass	0–2	3–4	5–6	≥7
Ragweed	0–3	4–9	10–16	≥17
Mug wort	0–6	7–15	16–27	≥28
Japanese hop	0–9	10–29	30–62	≥63

Unit is grain/m^3.

among the cities as well as reversely find his/her hazardous cities and periods based on the personal symptom history (**Fig. 2**).

- Pros: It can be used as a preliminary predictor for pollen risks.
- Cons: It is an average over certain past dates (up to 2 decades) so daily changing weather is not of concern. A calendar developed for a region represents the specific region where the data were collected, having the spatial distribution not readily presented.

FORECAST MODEL

Daily pollen concentration is highly dependent on weather conditions such as air temperature, relative humidity, solar radiation, and precipitation. Diagnostic models, developed from the observed data, can predict daily pollen concentration using the daily weather forecast (**Box 1**).

Regional Regression Model

Regional pollen risk forecast using regression models is performed in 3 steps as in **Box 1**.[30] KMA developed monthly pollen concentration models and provided trees/weeds pollen risks in spring (April and May)/autumn (September and October) (**Fig. 3**A). Selected weather variables are daily air temperature, temperature range, relative humidity, wind speed, precipitation hours, total precipitation, and 7-day accumulated sunshine hours. Using the pollen concentration, estimated from the regression models, risk grade was determined and daily risk levels were provided. Evaluation during the 2010 to 2011 period over the 6 regions showed an accuracy range from 31% to 100% (mean: 57.4%).

- Pros: The pollen risk forecast reflects daily weather conditions by assimilating output from the operational numerical weather forecasts.
- Cons: Models are developed for individual observational sites so that regional distribution and differences are not considered.

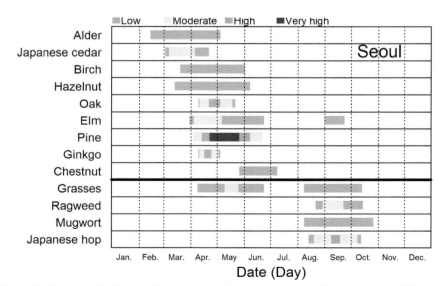

Fig. 2. Pollen calendar for Seoul, Korea, based on the updated observations in 2020.

> **Box 1**
> **Procedures of the development of the pollen risk forecast model using regression analysis**
>
> ① Find weather variables that affect pollen variability.
>
> ② Develop regression models for pollen concentration using the weather variables.
>
> ③ Estimate pollen concentration from the model and determine the pollen risk based on the concentration.

Probability-Regression Model

This is a unified model based on the analysis of probability distribution.[31] Simple regression models were developed from the data of individual sites and were able to predict specific sites. For the development of a nationwide service for pollen risks, it is needed to develop a unified model for pollen prediction that explains the weather conditions, which is commonly observed during the pollen outbreak. The find weather variables step ①-1 of **Box 2** is followed by 2 additional sub-steps: ①-2 fitting the histogram of pollen concentration by weather conditions to Weibull probability density function (PDF) and ①-3 calculating the daily probability of pollen appearance. The daily probability is then assimilated into the ② regression modeling and ③ risk estimation (see **Box 2**).

The PDF-regression model was developed using the daily weather variables (air temperature, degree-days, daily temperature range, relative humidity, wind speed, 7-day accumulated sunshine hours) and daily pollen concentration of oak and Japanese hop from 1997 to 2009 (**Fig. 3B**). Daily pollen concentration is represented as a histogram according to each weather variable. The histogram is the sum of probability of pollen appearance at a specific weather event and it is fitted to Weibull PDF. In other words, the PDF represents the probability of pollen observation by each weather variable. Then, regression models were developed using the PDFs of individual

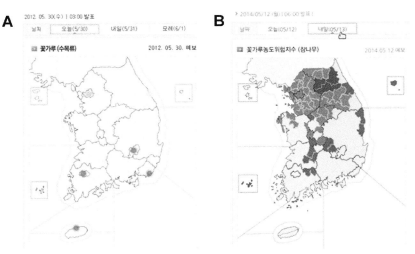

Fig. 3. (a) Regional pollen risk forecast based on the regional regression models in 2012 (b) National web service of pollen risk distribution by KMA using the PDF-regression model in 2014. *From* Korea Meteorological Administration. Available at: www.kma.go.kr Accessed 2012 and 2014. With permission.

Box 2
Procedures for the development of the pollen risk forecast model using probability density function and regression analysis

① -1 Find weather variables → ①-2 Fit the daily pollen probability into the Weibull probability density function → ①-3 Calculate daily pollen probability.

② Perform regression analysis.

③ Calculate pollen concentration and determine the risk grade from the concentration.

---

weather variables as independent ones and pollen concentration at all observational sites as the dependent one. Daily risk level was determined according to the risk grade standard. The model was validated using the observed data from 2010 to 2012. During the major pollen seasons of April and May for oak trees and September and October for Japanese hop, the index of agreement (IOA) between the model and observation was 70.8% and 90.3%, respectively—a large improvement from 60.4% and 78.1% of the original regional regression models.

- Pros: The regional regression models were simplified in the PDF-regression model, which is also able to predict the nationwide distribution of pollen risks using the operational numerical weather forecast because of its sole dependence on weather conditions.
- Cons: Other than weather conditions such as vegetation distribution and the physiologic difference is not reflected. Therefore the regional and yearly differences are excluded from the analysis and forecast. Also, despite the high IOA in pollen allergy risks, the pollen concentration was underestimated in general. The simulated length of pollen season and the dynamic fluctuation of pollen concentration such as daily maximum pollen concentration were suboptimal.

Probability-Machine Learning Model

The probability-regression model of the previous section failed to simulate peaks in the daily forecast and underestimated overall daily pollen concentration (**Box 3**). It was mainly caused by the characteristics of the dataset utilized in the model development of a high number of low concentration days. Additionally, the relationship between weather conditions and pollen concentration is not linear. To solve these problems, the probability of pollen appearance is estimated from weather data before machine learning models are programmed to predict pollen concentration (see **Box 3**). Additionally, to prevent over-fitting of the Deep Neural Network (DNN) model to the training data and underestimate the concentration, the bootstrap aggregating-type ensemble model was developed.[32] Nine stations with sufficient data during 2007 to

---

Box 3
Procedures of the development of pollen risk forecast model using probability density function and machine learning technique

① Find the probability of pollen appearance based on weather variables

② Train up machine learning models (eg, deep neural network, Random Forest) by the probability

③ Estimate pollen concentration and determine its risk level

2014 were selected for the training data. Because there are too many dates with a mild grade, the training set was re-composed as mild—the lowest grade—and non-mild grades equally by changing sampling frequency: mild 7%, moderate 80%, severe 90%, and extreme 100%. Several weather input variables were transformed into the daily probability of pollen appearance. The structure of the DNN model was determined through many kinds of experiments. The developed model was evaluated using the 9 station data during 2015 to 2016. Mean absolute percentage error (MAPE) of the pollen concentration was 5.6% to 4.5% and mean accuracy for the extreme grade was 45.5%, which was a great improvement from 28.4% of the regional regression models. Periods of pollen season, when taking action against pollen allergy is needed, are compared by the dates of start and end of the season. During the evaluation period, the DNN model outperformed the regression models: deviations from the observed start/end of the season were 4 to 8/7 to 11 days and 13 to 26/29 to 36 days by the DNN and regression models, respectively. The DNN models have been implemented as an operational service in KMA since 2017.

- Pros: Accuracy is higher than in conventional models. Machine learning models make the most use of the observed data.
- Cons: It is a black-box model. Developed models have not considered the long-term vegetation changes nor regional and yearly variations in pollen production so that they need a periodic update with continued observation. As with the pollen types with a lower concentration, machine learning models are equally disadvantageous as other conventional models. Only the pollen types observed commonly and frequently are applicable for practical modeling.

Pollen Dispersal Model

Detailed mid- and long-range pollen forecast can be achieved by simulating dissemination-transportation-deposition with dispersal models like the Asian dust forecast. Pollen dispersal and risk models can be developed over a large area based on vegetation distribution and phenological flowering models even though the insufficient observational data for probability-regression or machine learning models. The birch and the Japanese cedar forecast of Finland and Japan, respectively, incorporated dispersal forecast models.[26,38–42]

CMAQ, developed by the US Environmental Protection Agency, was used as the basic modeling system. The UK Met office's Unified Model Local Data Assimilation and Prediction System, one of KMA's operational numerical weather prediction systems, was assimilated as the input. The behavior of pollen grains was simulated as an aerosol with the property of chemically inactive coarse particles. Moreover, a module for pollen emission and data processing was newly developed.

The Forestry Geographic Information System (FGIS) tree stand data (1:5000) was provided by the Korea Forest Service. Gridded pollen emission was estimated from the oak tree distribution, which is converted from the FGIS coverage map of oak trees according to the grid resolution of the numerical weather forecast. The key components of the emission model were flowering period and yearly total pollen production. In the emission model, daily pollen release was determined from the Weibull PDF model, which was tuned to produce yearly total pollen concentration of 85,000 grains m^{-3}, which was observed in 2-year intensive observation at the Gwangneung oak forest. For the evaluation of the model, temporal changes in the spatial distribution of the pollen emission were investigated. Because the daily pollen concentration model is driven by degree-days, the shift of emission place from southern plain to northern mountain areas was simulated as expected (**Fig. 4**). However, the temporal patterns

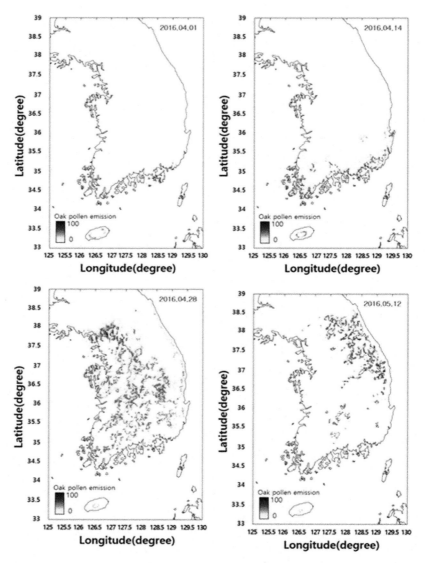

Fig. 4. Temporal changes in national pollen emission estimated by the model according to degree-days. (source: unpublished data).

of simulated daily concentrations in 2016 were earlier or later than the observation depending on the station. The estimated pollen season by the DNN model was also inconsistently matched with the observation. Major shortcomings of the dispersal model existed within the emission model such as the uncertainty of the vegetation distribution and neglected genetic diversity of the oak trees.

- Pros: It is possible to integrate a variety of data including meteorology, phenology, and remote sensing. Dispersal models can produce background information against new and novel pollen using the basic knowledge of plant physiology without sufficient direct observation.

- Cons: Pollen production and emission are highly affected by plant phenology (flowering), dispersal meteorology, and hourly emission just like the regional regression model. It is difficult to improve the accuracy of component data/models such as vegetation distribution for source area, plant phenology for the flowering period, and physical behavior of pollen grains for hourly dispersal.

FURTHER RESEARCH

Research items identified to improve operational pollen allergy models and services in KMA are as follows:

Year-Over-Year Variation Model of Pollen Concentration

As described before, the operational KMA pollen allergy forecast models were developed from the relationship between daily weather conditions and pollen concentration using the modeling methods of the probability distribution, statistical regression, and deep neural network. Conventional models for pollen concentration forecasts like these cannot answer to year-over-year variation because they reflect the relationship of daily weather and pollen only. In other words, the same date with the same daily weather conditions will produce the same concentration of pollen. However, the long-term observation shows a great variation of yearly total pollen concentration. Elements that affect the yearly variation of tree pollen can be the conditions for vegetative growth of the previous year, for production of over-wintering dormant buds, and for over-wintering itself.

To predict the regional difference of yearly pollen concentration it is needed to analyze and model the differences using long-term observed data (**Box 4**).

Analysis of Year-Over-Year Variation of Oak Pollen

Oak pollen, known to exist all around Korea with a high variation over regions and years, was studied to develop a prediction model for yearly pollen concentration using monthly weather data from 1 year before. Daily pollen concentration was observed using Burkard traps at 9 stations in Korea from 1998 to 2019. Yearly total from each station was transformed into a common logarithm (Iconc). Selected weather data were daily mean or total at the nearest KMA stations (ASOS or AWS). They were processed as monthly mean air temperature and wind speed and monthly total precipitation and then standardized using their mean and standard deviations. Monthly weather data from January to April were regarded as the previous year's data. Data from 1998 to 2017 were used in the model development and 2018 to 2019 data in the validation.

A t-test was performed to determine the monthly weather elements on yearly pollen. From each station, years with high and low 20% of yearly total concentration were selected and the differences in monthly (1–12) mean temperature (T), mean wind speed (W), and total precipitation (P) were compared using the t-test analysis.

Box 4
Procedures for the development of a prediction model of yearly total pollen

① Input data processing for modeling: monthly total pollen concentration and weather conditions of the previous year

② Model development: regression analysis

③ Predicted variable: yearly total pollen concentration

A forecasting model for yearly total pollen concentration was developed through regression analysis. Seven independent variables were selected based on the t-test analysis: T4 (April temperature) and P8 (August precipitation) had negative and T8, T10, W6, W8, and P12 had positive coefficients. The total pollen concentration of the previous year (Iconc1), in addition to the monthly weather variables, were considered as the independent variables to account for regional differences in vegetational distribution. The regression model with these eight selected variables explained 41% of the yearly variation of total pollen ($R^2 = 0.41$). It was evaluated using the data from 2018 to 2019. Its RMSE, MAE, ME, and R^2 were 0.28, 0.22, −0.0073, and 0.24, respectively.

Most of the previous studies regarding long-term changes in pollen concentration emphasized the long-term increase/decrease of the concentration disregarding weather conditions or the future projection based on climate change scenarios. In addition, short-term pollen forecasting models cannot reflect the nature of yearly fluctuation of pollens. A yearly variation model of the current study can be integrated with the daily pollen forecast model to improve the daily forecast's accuracy.

- Pros: Yearly pollen concentration is predicted based on the previous year's plant growth. Information on yearly pollen concentration can be provided prior to the pollen season.
- Cons: It is difficult to analyze the biological meaning of the model's parameters. Regional deviations in phenology observed at the early season of the year need to be reflected in the model for improved accuracy.

Climate Change and Impact Prediction

Climate change due to the increase in atmospheric CO_2 affects plant physiology and ecology.

Weeds: common ragweed

Common ragweed is small and takes a short amount of time from seeding to flowering; therefore, conducting CO_2 enrichment experiments is feasible using climate chambers. Ziska and Caulfield[43] reported the changes in ragweed pollen production at current (370 ppm) and future (600 ppm) as 131% and 320% increase, respectively, from pre-industrial CO_2 concentration (280 ppm), based on the climate chamber experiments. Singer and colleagues[44] analyzed the changes in allergenic protein Amb a1 at the current concentration from the pre-industrial, and at the future from the current as an x1.8 and x1.6 increase, respectively. In Korea, Choi and colleagues[45] performed CO_2 concentration experiments using climate chambers and on-site difference between urban and suburban sites. The chamber experiments showed a 230% and 272% increase of Amb a1 concentration under two future CO_2 scenarios (600 ppm and 1000 ppm) from the current (380 ppm). At the urban and suburban sites, the mean observed CO_2 concentration was 440 ppm and 320 ppm, respectively. At the urban site, the mean Amb a1 concentration of 20.4 ng/mL was higher than 16.3 ng/mL at the suburban site; although, the difference was statistically insignificant.

Trees: oak

Pollen production experiments of trees by CO_2 concentration are limited by canopy size and long-time exposure. Kim and colleagues[46] used open-top CO_2 chambers (OTC) to maintain CO_2 concentrations at ambient (~400 ppm), x1.4 (~560 ppm), and x1.8 (~720 ppm) for more than 7 years. The production of pollen grains and allergen Que a1 by sawtooth oak trees under the chambers was quantitatively assessed. Total pollen counts per tree of the x1.4 and x1.8 treatments showed a significant increase of 353% and 1299%, respectively, from the ambient conditions. Allergenic protein contents at the x1.4 and x1.8 treatments also showed significant increase of 12% and 11%, respectively.

Considering several aspects of the CO_2 experiments altogether, the elevated CO_2 concentration by the future change of the climate, will surely bring us a higher plant growth and more pollen production. Concentration of allergens from trees and weeds is predicted to increase by higher CO_2 concentration, despite some experimental results, without a statistical significance. In other words, under the future higher CO_2 concentration, people will be exposed to higher allergen levels; therefore, keep-watching and well-preparedness on pollen concentration and patient reaction are needed. However, the actual level of elevated allergy risks is hard to be predicted due to the underlying plant physiology and ecology in the real world resulting from complex impacts of environment change, including air temperature, rainfall, soil nutrition, and changing flowering periods.

DISCUSSION

Pollen allergy risk information and KMA models are summarized in **Table 2**. The meta data are important in the operation of the observational network. During the network funding sources transition from KAPARD to KMA, several stations missed the observation during that period (2006). In 2018, the observational stations were relocated around the KMA's observational fields around the country. Detailed information along with the meta data are described in the technical note of NIMS/KMA. Meta

Table 2
Observational data and models in relation to pollen allergy in Korea Meteorological Administration (KMA)

Model	Species/ Identification Group	Station	Data Period	Interval/ Forecast	Service Year/ Stations (Regions)
		Model Development		**Operational Service by KMA**	
Observation	21 (2019–)	12	1997–	Daily (near realtime data only)/NA	2019/2
Pollen Calendar v2008	17	6	1997–2007	10 days/1 y	2008/6
v2010	17	6	1997–2009	10 days/1 y	2010/6
v2019	13	8	2007–2017	Daily/1 y	2019/8
GLM	3	6(7)	2001–2006 (1997–2009)	Daily/2 d	2008 (2011)/6(7)
PDF-GLM	3	7	1997–2009	Daily/2 d	2014/National
PDF-DNN	2	9	2007–2014	Daily/2 d	2017/National
Pollen Dispersal	Oak	1	2015–2016	Daily/2 d	NA/National
Yearly variation	Oak	9	1998–2017	Yearly/1 y	NA/National
CO_2 impact	Oak		2016	NA/ 30–50 y	NA/NA

Abbreviations: DNN, deep neural network; GLM, general linear model; NA, not applicable; PDF, probability density function.

information, such as site relocation and data loss, should be considered in the data analysis for modeling.[33]

By continuing pollen observation, the pollen calendar can be developed and utilized for patient consultation. The accumulated long-term observation data allow the use of probability distribution models to quantitatively estimate daily pollen risks. Individual patients are able to match their own risk levels by comparing their historical symptom diary with the daily risk level obtained by the regional pollen calendar. Integrating information technology (IT) into the pollen calendar would allow the development of a personalized outdoor activity calendar using the symptom diary on their own.

Short-term forecast of pollen allergy using daily weather data was best performed by machine learning methods, in terms of technical advancement and accuracy. In addition, the yearly pollen risk level would be provided if the yearly total pollen concentration model was operated before the pollen season. If long-range transport is challenging, dispersal models can be implemented. However, because most pollens in Korea originate from local flora, the accuracy of the forecast depends on vegetation distribution models, plant phenology, and plant physiology. Conversely, dispersal models have limited functionality. All biometeorological information regarding human health are expected to help increase the people's quality of life. The purpose of these services is to provide adequate pollen allergy information based on field observation. The observational network should be endlessly upgraded, incorporating new technology, such as automatic observation, to maintain its consistency by network expansion. Another important aspect of pollen risk forecast is the relationship between pollen count and the allergic patients' symptom level. Regional difference and temporal changes are essential subjects for the preparedness against climate change.

CLINICS CARE POINTS

- Pollen allergy calendar: If we carefully examine the personal allergic symptom diary with pollen calendar, it will be possible to provide personalized outdoor activity calendar and prescription for the patient.
- Pollen risk forecast: In addition to the pollen calendar, a daily forecast on pollen allergy risks by weather service agencies will provide a more detailed day-to-day risk information.
- Symptom index study: The links between pollen counts and symptom index by allergy patients are highly affected by the characteristics of pollinating plants and regional climate. It should be locally studied considering regional differences.

ACKNOWLEDGMENTS

This work was funded by the Korea Meteorological Administration Research and Development Program "Advanced Research on Biometeorology and Industrial Meteorology" under Grant number (KMA2018-00620).

DISCLOSURE

The authors have nothing to disclose.

REFERENCES

1. Fuhrman C, Sarter H, Thibaudon M, et al. Short-term effect of pollen exposure on antiallergic drug consumption. Ann Allergy Asthma Immunol 2007;99:225–31.

2. Darrow LA, Hess J, Rogers CA, et al. Ambient pollen concentrations and emergency department visits for asthma and wheeze. J Allergy Clin Immunol 2012; 130:630–8.
3. D'Amato G, Holgate ST, Pawankar R, et al. Meteorological conditions, climate change, new emerging factors, and asthma and related allergic disorders. A statement of the World Allergy Organization. World Allergy Organ J 2015;8:25.
4. Kim S-H, Park H-S, Jang J-Y. Impact of meteorological variation on hospital visits of patients with tree pollen allergy. BMC Public Health 2011;11:890.
5. Kim HY, Kwon EB, Baek JH, et al. Prevalence and comorbidity of allergic diseases in preschool children. Korean J Pediatr 2013;56:338–42.
6. Ito K, Weinberger KR, Robinson GS, et al. The associations between daily spring pollen counts, over-the-counter allergy medication sales, and asthma syndrome emergency department visits in New York City, 2002-2012. Environ Health 2015;14:71.
7. Ariano R, Berra D, Chiodini E, et al. Ragweed allergy: pollen count and sensitization and allergy prevalence in two Italian allergy centers. Allergy Rhinol (Providence) 2015;6:177–83.
8. Park HJ, Lim HS, Park KH, et al. Changes in allergen sensitization over the last 30 years in Korea respiratory allergic patients: a single-center. Allergy Asthma Immunol Res 2014;6:434–43.
9. IQVIA. National allergy forecast and info about allergies. 2020. Available at: https://www.pollen.com/. Accessed April 16, 2020.
10. WeatherBug: Local allergy forecasts and pollen count reports. Available at: https://www.weatherbug.com/life/pollen/. Accessed April 16, 2020.
11. Met Office: Pollen forecast. Available at: https://www.metoffice.gov.uk/warnings-and-advice/seasonal-advice/pollen-forecast/. Accessed April 16, 2020.
12. Zyrtec: App and allergy forecast tool. Available at: https://www.zyrtec.com/allergy-forecast-tools-apps/. Accessed April 16, 2020.
13. Galan C, Carinanos P, Garcia-Mozo H, et al. Model for forecasting *Olea europaea* L. airborne pollen in south-west Andalusia, Spain. Int J Biometeorol 2001;45: 59–63.
14. De Weger LA, Beerthuizen T, Hiemstra PS, et al. Development and validation of a 5-day-ahead hay fever forecast for patients with grass-pollen-induced allergic rhinitis. Int J Biometeorol 2014;58:1047–55.
15. Driessen MNBM, Van Herpen RMA, Moelands RPM, et al. Prediction of the start of the grass pollen season for the western part of the Netherlands. Grana 1989;28: 37–44.
16. Emberlin J, Mullins J, Corden J, et al. Regional variations in grass pollen seasons in the UK, long-term trends and forecast models. Clin Exp Allergy 1999;29: 347–56.
17. Galan C, Emberlin J, Dominguez E, et al. A comparative analysis of daily variations in the Gramineae pollen counts at Cordoba, Spain and London, UK. Grana 1995;34:189–98.
18. Jato V, Rodriguez-Rajo FJ, Alcazar P, et al. May the definition of pollen season influence aerobiological results? Aerobiologia 2006;22:13–25.
19. Khwarahm N, Dash J, Atkinson PM, et al. Exploring the spatio-temporal relationship between two key aeroallergens and meteorological variables in the United Kingdom. Int J Biometeorol 2014;58:529–45.
20. Kim JH, Oh JW, Lee HB, et al. Evaluation of the association of vegetation of allergenic plants and pollinosis with meteorological changes. Allergy Asthma Respir Dis 2014;2:48–58 [in Korean with English abstract].

21. Larsson KA. Prediction of the pollen season with a cumulated activity method. Grana 1993;32:111–4.

22. Lee HR, Kim KR, Choi YJ, et al. Meteorological impact on daily concentration of pollen in Korea. Korean J Agr and Forest Meteorol 2012;14:99–107 [in Korean with English abstract].

23. Norris-Hill J. The modeling of daily Poaceae pollen concentrations. Grana 1995; 34:182–8.

24. Sabariego S, Cuesta P, Fernandez-Gonzalez F, et al. Models for forecasting airborne Cupressaceae pollen levels in Central Spain. Int J Biometeorol 2012; 56:253–8.

25. Subiza J, Masiello JM, Subiza JL, et al. Prediction of annual variations in atmospheric concentrations of grass pollen. A method based on meteorological factors and grain crop estimates. Clin Exp Allergy 1992;22:540–6.

26. Toro FJ, Recio M, Trigo MM, et al. Predictive models in aerobiology: data transformation. Aerobiologia 1998;14:179–84.

27. Efstathiou C, Isukapalli S, Georgopoulos P. A mechanistic modeling system for estimating largescale emissions and transport of pollen and co-allergens. Atmos Environ 2011;45:2260–76.

28. Helbig N, Vogel B, Vogel H, et al. Numerical modelling of pollen dispersion on the regional scale. Aerobiologia 2004;20:3–19.

29. Sofiev M, Siljamo P, Ranta H, et al. A numerical model of birch pollen emission and dispersion in the atmosphere. Description of emission module. Int J Biometeorol 2013;57:45–58.

30. Kim KR, Park KJ, Lee HR, et al. Development and evaluation of the forecast models for daily pollen allergy. Korean J Agr and Forest Meteorol 2012;14: 265–8 [in Korean with English abstract].

31. Kim KR, Kim M, Choe H-S, et al. A biology-driven receptor model for daily pollen allergy risk in Korea based on Weibull probability density function. Int J Biometeorol 2017;61:259–72.

32. Seo YA, Kim KR, Cho C, et al. Deep neural network-based concentration model for oak pollen allergy warning in South Korea. Allergy Asthma Immunol Res 2020; 12:149–63.

33. Han MJ, Kim MW, Cho C, et al. Operators' technical note on pollen monitoring network. Seogwipo-si, Republic of Korea: National Institute of Meteorological Sciences (NIMS); NIMS 11-1360620-000155-01 2019. p. 74. [in Korean].

34. Oh J-W, Lee H-B, Kang I-J, et al. The revised edition of Korean calendar for allergenic pollens. Allergy Asthma Immunol Res 2012;4:5–11.

35. Park K-J, Kim H-A, Kim KR, et al. Characteristics of regional distribution of pollen concentration in Korean Peninsula. Korean J Agr and Forest Meteorol 2008;10: 167–76 [in Korean with English abstract].

36. AAAAI. Reading the NAB pollen count charts. Available at: https://www.aaaai. org/global/nab-pollen-counts/reading-the-charts/. Accessed April 17, 2020.

37. Shin J-Y, Han MJ, Cho C, et al. Allergenic pollen calendar in Korea based on probability distribution models and up-to-date observations. Allergy Asthma Immunol Res 2020;12:259–73.

38. Siljamo P, Sofev M, Filatova E, et al. A numerical model of birch pollen emission and dispersion in the atmosphere. Model evaluation and sensitivity analysis. Int J Biometeorol 2013;57:125–36.

39. Vogel H, Pauling A, Vogel B. Numerical simulation of birch pollen dispersion with an operational weather forecast system. Int J Biometeorol 2008;52:805–14.

40. Suzuki M, Sasaki A, Tonouchi M, Yamamoto C. Long term pollen dispersion forecast model for Japanese cedar and cypress. 92nd American Meteorological Society Annual Meeting, New Orleans, LA, 22-26 January, 2012.

41. Lim YK, Kim KR, Cho C, et al. Development of an oak pollen emission and transport modeling framework in South Korea. Atmosphere 2015;25:221–33 [in Korean with English abstract].

42. Kim T-H, Seo YA, Kim KR, et al. Improvement and evaluation of emission formulas in UM-CMAQ-Pollen model. Atmosphere 2019;29:1–12 [in Korean with English abstract].

43. Ziska LH, Caulfield FA. Rising CO_2 and pollen production of common ragweed (*Ambrosia artemisiifolia*), a known allergy-inducing species: implications for public health. Aust J Plant Physiol 2000;27:893–8.

44. Singer BD, Ziska LH, Frenz DA, et al. Increasing Amb a 1 content in common ragweed (*Ambrosia artemisiifolia*) pollen as a function of rising atmospheric CO_2 concentration. Funct Plant Biol 2005;32:667–70.

45. Choi Y-J, Oh H-R, Oh J-W, et al. Chamber and field studies demonstrate differential Amb a 1 contents in common ragweed depending on CO_2 levels. Allergy Asthma Immunol Res 2018;10:278–82.

46. Kim KR, Oh J-W, Woo S-Y, et al. Does the increase in ambient CO_2 concentration elevate allergy risks posed by oak pollen? Int J Biometeorol 2018;62:1587–94.

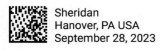